The Healthy Clothes Closet

Ten Principles for a Woman's Wardrobe

Jean Marie Smith, N.D.

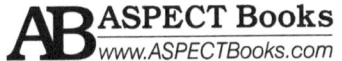

World rights reserved. This book or any portion thereof may not be copied or reproduced in any form or manner whatever, except as provided by law, without the written permission of the publisher, except by a reviewer who may quote brief passages in a review.

The author assumes full responsibility for the accuracy of all facts and quotations as cited in this book. The opinions expressed in this book are the author's personal views and interpretations, and do not necessarily reflect those of the publisher.

This book is provided with the understanding that the publisher is not engaged in giving spiritual, legal, medical, or other professional advice. If authoritative advice is needed, the reader should seek the counsel of a competent professional.

Copyright © 2018 Jean Marie Smith, N.D.
Copyright © 2018 ASPECT Books, Inc.
ISBN-13: 978-1-4796-0483-0 (Paperback)
Library of Congress Control Number: 2018908383

Amplified Bible (AMP): Copyright© 2015 by The Lockman Foundation. All rights reserved.

Amplified Bible, Classic Edition (AMPC): Copyright© 1954,1958,1962,1964,1965,1987 by The Lockman Foundation.

Common English Bible (CEB): Copyright© 2011 by Common English Bible.

King James Version (KJV): Public Domain.

New International Version (NIV): Holy Bible, New International Version®, NIV® Copyright© 1973, 1978, 1984, 2011 by Biblica, Inc.® Used by permission. All rights reserved worldwide.

New King James Version (NKJV): Scripture taken from the New King James Version®. Copyright© 1982 by Thomas Nelson. Used by permission. All rights reserved.

Living Bible (TLV): The Living Bible copyright© 1971 by Tyndale House Foundation. Used by permission of Tyndale House Publishers Inc., Carol Stream, Illinois 60188. All rights reserved.

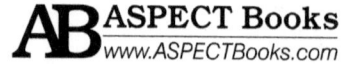

Acknowledgments

I give all glory to our wonderful Heavenly Father and our dearest Lord and Savior Jesus Christ. They have been so faithful in answering my prayers to send a "writing angel" to guide me on every page.

I am also grateful for the love and support of my precious husband, David. His encouragement and support have made God's calling possible.

Dedication

This book is dedicated to you, dear reader. May these principles and applications help fulfill our kind Lord's desire for you: "Beloved, I pray that you may prosper in all things and be in health, just as your soul prospers" (3 John 2, NKJV).

Contents

Introduction 1

Chapter One   Protection from the Sun 3

Chapter Two   Keep Cool with Proper Clothing 13

Chapter Three Keep Warm with Adequate Clothing 22

Chapter Four   Dressing for Healthful Circulation 28

Chapter Five   Honor Your Feminine Organs 36

Chapter Six   Footwear that "Kills" Your Feet 45

Chapter Seven Posture and Purses 52

Chapter Eight Fabrics for Health 62

Chapter Nine   Cleanliness and Toxins 74

Chapter Ten   Complexion, Colors and Cosmetics 82

Conclusion 90

Bibliography 91

Introduction

The oft-repeated question, "What shall we wear?" (Matthew 6:31), may seem to be only a contemporary concern of women. Yet it was just as much an issue over two thousand years ago, when Jesus Christ gave His life-changing Sermon on the Mount.

Wardrobe planning and clothing choices can have different motivations for different women, including fashion expression, job performance and advancement, social acceptance and attraction of the opposite sex. Nonetheless, all women can be benefitted by learning principles of health in relation to clothing selection.

Many individuals are not aware of the cause-and-effect relationship between genetics, lifestyle and health. Many of us do not understand the beautiful systems of our bodies that our wonderful Creator has made, and how to respectfully take care of ourselves in such a way as to prevent much of the illness that plagues humanity, including how we dress.

"Disease never comes without a cause. The way is prepared, and disease invited, by disregard of the laws of health. Many suffer in consequence of the transgression of their parents. While they are not responsible for what their parents have done, it is nevertheless their duty to ascertain what are and what are not violations of the laws of health. They should avoid the wrong habits of their parents and, by correct living, place themselves in better conditions.

"The greater number, however, suffer because of their own wrong course of action. They disregard the principles of health by their habits of eating, drinking, dressing, and working. Their transgression of nature's laws produces the sure result; and when sickness comes upon them, many do not credit their suffering to the true cause, but murmur against God because of their afflictions. But God is not responsible for the suffering that follows disregard of natural law."[1]

"The only hope of better things is in the education of the people in right principles. Let physicians teach the people that restorative power is not in drugs, but in nature. Disease is an effort of nature to free the system from conditions that result from a violation of the laws of health. In case of sickness, the cause should be ascertained. Unhealthful conditions should be changed, wrong habits corrected. Then nature is to be assisted in her effort to expel impurities and to re-establish right conditions in the system."[2]

In the pages that follow, we will explore ten principles of healthful dress. Using the Ten Commandments from Exodus 20:1–17 as the framework, we will discuss physical applications for clothing and health from the commandments' far-reaching implications.

> *"That you may remember and do all My commandments*
> *and be holy to your God."*
> *Numbers 15:40, AMPC*

---

[1] White, E. G. (1905). *The Ministry of Healing*. Mountain View, CA: Pacific Press Publishing Association, 234.
[2] Ibid, 127.

CHAPTER ONE

Protection from the Sun

The First Commandment

*"I am the L*ORD *your God, who brought you out of the land of Egypt, out of the house of bondage. You shall have no other gods before Me."*
Exodus 20: 2, 3, NKJV

Principle

Clothing assists in protection from the damage of sun "worship."

The biblical record of Creation states that "God made the two great lights—the greater light (the sun) to rule the day and the lesser light (the moon) to rule the night . . . God saw that it was good (fitting, pleasant) and He approved it" (Genesis 1:16, 18, AMPC). Sunlight certainly is good, for it is the source of our planet's light, warmth and energy. We are dependent upon sunlight for the photosynthesized energy stored in plant foods, which provide our caloric intake from carbohydrates, protein and fats.[3]

Sunlight has numerous health benefits. Its ultraviolet light increases the body's resistance to infections by increasing the lymphocytes and phagocytic index.[4] Sunlight's effects are similar to exercise, in that it can decrease blood pressure, resting heart and

---

[3] Kime, Zane R. (1980). *Sunlight Could Save Your Life.* Penryn, CA: World Health Publications, 21.

[4] Ibid, 31.

respiratory rates, and blood glucose. Simultaneously, it can increase cardiac output, oxygenation of the blood, glycogen stores in the liver, stress tolerance and energy, endurance and muscular strength.[5]

Sunshine entering unshaded eyes increases seratonin production, which can help depression and fatigue. Sunlight can also increase hormonal levels of melatonin at night, which aids in sleep quality.[6] A study published in 2017 highlighted not only the well-known fact that sunshine on exposed skin increases serum vitamin D levels, but also that it lowers total cholesterol levels, lowering both HDL and LDL cholesterol.[7]

The previous paragraph, listing the positive effects of sunlight upon our health, certainly contrasts with the abundance of public warnings against unprotected sun exposure to help prevent skin cancer and other health risks. The Scriptures offer us an important principle to help with a moderate approach. "Every athlete who goes into training conducts himself temperately and restricts himself in all things" (1 Corinthians 9:25, AMPC). "True temperance teaches us to abstain entirely from that which is injurious, and to use healthful and nutritious articles judiciously."[8] Regarding sunlight, its intelligent use can contribute to overall health; however, indiscriminate exposure will certainly pose a health risk. In fact, Dr. Zane Kime states that "unless one has a proper diet, sunlight has an ill effect on the skin . . . Sunbathing is dangerous for those who are on the standard high-fat American diet or do not get

---

[5] Ibid, 46.

[6] Nedley, Neil, (2001) *Depression: The Way Out.* Ardmore, OK: Nedley Publishing, 88.

[7] Sorenson, Marc, "Sun Exposure and Vitamin D Reduce Cholesterol Levels," Sunlight Institute. http://sunlightinstitute.org/sun-exposure-vitamin-d-cholesterol/

[8] White, Ellen G., *The Review and Herald,* September 23, 1884 par. 5

an abundance of vegetables, whole grains, and fresh fruit."[9]

There are 2 main types of ultraviolet (UV) rays that damage our skin. Both types can cause skin cancer: UVB, which is responsible for majority of sunburns, and UVA, which penetrates deep into the skin, causing aging but contributes much less towards sunburn. "Sunburn is a clear sign that the DNA in your skin cells has been damaged by too much UV radiation. Getting sunburn, just once every 2 years, can triple your risk of melanoma skin cancer."[10]

Sunlight has been found to be beneficial, however, with the prevention and survival rates of melanoma patients. "Several studies have confirmed that appropriate sun exposure actually helps *prevent* skin cancer. In fact, melanoma occurrence has been found to *decrease* with greater sun exposure, and can be increased by sunscreens. One such study revealed that melanoma patients who had higher levels of sun exposure were less likely to die than other melanoma patients, and patients who already had melanoma and got a lot of sun exposure were prone to a less aggressive tumor type. Another Italian study, published in the *European Journal of Cancer* in June 2008, also confirms and supports earlier studies showing improved survival rates in melanoma patients who were exposed to sunlight more frequently in the time before their melanoma was diagnosed. Also, melanoma is actually more common in indoor workers than in outdoor workers, and is more common on regions of your body that are not exposed to the sun at all. UVB radiation has been found to delay the appearance of melanoma if you are

---

[9] Kime, 117.

[10] Cancer Research UK, "How the Sun and UV Cause Cancer," Cancer Research UK. http://www.cancerresearchuk.org/about-cancer/causes-of-cancer/sun-uv-and-cancer/how-the-sun-and-uv-cause-cancer

genetically predisposed or prone to skin cancer."[11]

An adequate amount of sunlight on exposed skin (face and arms) is approximately 30 minutes a day, three times a week for most light-skinned individuals, with longer time needed for those with darker skin. Gradual increase in sun exposure is wise for those just starting, beginning with five minutes.[12] Consideration needs to be given to the increased intensity of sunlight when reflected from water or sand, or when submerged under water, with decreased time to prevent burning.[13] Time outdoors in the sunshine for longer periods requires adequate clothing coverage.

"Clothing is a simple, effective sun protection tool that shades the skin from ultraviolet A (UVA), or long wave, and ultraviolet B (UVB), or short wave, rays. It provides a physical block that doesn't wash or wear off. Long-sleeved shirts and pants, hats with broad brims and sunglasses are all effective forms of sun protective clothing."[14]

"Clothing is our first line of defense against the sun's harmful ultraviolet (UV) rays and protects us by absorbing or

---

[11] Mercola, Joseph, "Sun Can Actually Help Protect You Against Skin Cancer," Dr. Mercola's Health Articles.
https://articles.mercola.com/sites/articles/archive/2011/06/16/sun-can-protect-you-against-skin-cancer.aspx

[12] *Amazing Health Facts!* (2009). Roseville, CA: Amazing Facts, Inc., 25.

[13] UPF Clothing, "Sea and Sand Can Increase UV Radiation by 25%," UPF Clothing.
http://upfclothing.org/sea-sand-can-increase-uv-radiation-by-25/

[14] USCF Medical Center, "Protective Clothing for Skin Cancer Protection," USCF.
https://www.ucsfhealth.org/education/protective_clothing_for_skin_cancer_prevention/

blocking much of this radiation. The more skin you cover, the better. A long-sleeved shirt covers more skin than a t-shirt, especially if it has a high neckline or collar that shields the back of the neck. Likewise, long pants protect more skin than shorts . . . A wide-brimmed (3-inch or greater) hat covers places like the scalp where it is difficult to apply sunscreen or areas where people forget to apply sunscreen, including the tops of the ear and the back of the neck."[15]

Clothing coverage is a much safer option for sun protection than commercial sunscreen. The Environmental Working Group reports several common ingredients in sunscreens that are estrogenic hormone disruptors and were found to be present in breast milk. Additionally, some sunscreen ingredients used in adult and children's products have been found to contribute to high rates of skin allergies.[16]

The winter months also can pose a need for sun protection. "Many people forget about sun protection in cold weather venues. But ice and snow reflect about 80 percent of the sun's UV light, almost doubling the intensity of exposure. Both snow and strong wind can wear away sunscreen, reducing its effectiveness. Again, hats are important, and knitted winter hats made of high-tech, man-made materials will keep you comfortable as well as sun-

---

[15] Skin Cancer Foundation, "What You Need to Know About Clothing," Skin Cancer Foundation.
http://www.skincancer.org/prevention/sun-protection/clothing
[16] Environmental Working Group, "The Trouble With Ingredients in Sunscreens," EWG.
https://www.ewg.org/sunscreen/report/the-trouble-with-sunscreen-chemicals/#.WdV-CNEpBPY

protected."[17]

When choosing clothing for sun protection, it is important to consider the qualities of the fabrics. "Of course, you can have clothing over every square inch of your body, but if the sun goes right through it, it's not much use. Fabrics are made of tiny fibers woven or knitted together. Under a microscope, we can see lots of spaces between the fibers; UV can pass directly through these holes to reach the skin. The tighter the knit or weave, the smaller the holes and the less UV can get through. Twill, used to make tweeds or denim, is an example of a tightly woven fabric. Open weave fabrics provide much less protection.

"Fabrics can be made from many types of fibers, including cotton, wool, and nylon. Most fibers naturally absorb some UV radiation, and some have elastic threads that pull the fibers tightly together, reducing the spaces between the holes. Synthetic fibers such as polyester, lycra, nylon, and acrylic are more protective than bleached cottons, and shiny or lustrous semi-synthetic fabrics like rayon reflect more UV than do matte ones, such as linen, which tend to absorb rather than reflect UV. Finally, consider the fabric's weight and density—light, sheer silk gauze will provide far less UV protection than heavy cotton denim."[18]

Some additional factors for sun-safe clothing include:

---

[17] Skin Cancer Foundation, "Clothing: Our First Line of Defense," Skin Cancer Foundation. http://www.skincancer.org/prevention/sun-protection/clothing/clothing-our-first-line-of-defense

[18] Skin Cancer Foundation, "What Is Sun-Safe Clothing?," Skin Cancer Foundation. http://www.skincancer.org/prevention/sun-protection/clothing/protection

1. Buy garments that suit your purpose. You don't need a heavy work shirt for the beach, but a long-sleeved, tightly woven linen shirt can be both cool and sun-smart.

2. If you are buying elastic garments like leggings, make sure you purchase the right size—overstretching will lower the UPF rating.

3. Look for garments with a UPF of at least 30 so that you know you're getting effective sun protection.

4. Choose garments that cover more skin—there's no point in a high-UPF bikini. Instead, consider a rash guard or swim shirt. Made of lightweight, elastic materials like spandex, these athletic tops will cover your upper body without weighing you down.

5. You can also have beach skirts or sarongs ready for when you leave the water. Wash new garments made from cotton or cotton blends two or three times at least. This can often permanently raise the U.P.F. rating due to shrinkage of the spaces between the fibers.[19]

Sun-protective clothing, when chosen and used correctly, is the best form of sun protection.

One additional item of sun protection is sunglasses. Many beauty and fashion-conscious women believe an outdoor outfit is incomplete without sunglasses. Not only for reducing glare or wrinkles, there are health benefits from wearing sunglasses.

"After a long day at the beach, eyes may seem bloodshot, swollen, and light-sensitive. Sunburn of the eye, or photokeratitis, is one effect. It's also known as "snow blindness," as it happens to skiers, too. In severe cases, it can cause loss of vision for up to 48

---

[19] Ibid.

hours.

"It's not necessary to buy expensive sunglasses," says Paul Michelson, M.D., an ophthalmologist in La Jolla, Calif., and chairman of the Better Vision Institute, the medical advisory arm to The Vision Council. More important, he says, is to "choose a pair that offers protection from both U.V.A. and U.V.B. rays. Both types can damage vision."[20]

"The eyelid region is one of the most common sites for nonmelanoma skin cancers. In fact, skin cancers of the eyelid, including basal cell carcinoma (B.C.C.), squamous cell carcinoma (SCC), and melanoma, account for five to 10 percent of all skin cancers. Ninety five percent of these tumors are basal cell carcinomas or squamous cell carcinomas."[21]

In a study that examined "the effectiveness of 32 pairs of inexpensive sunglasses in filtering UVR, they found that all sunglasses studied transmitted less than two percent of UVB. Sunglasses were more effective in blocking UV than prescription eyeglasses, but moving the glasses a small distance from the forehead (further out on the nose) resulted in a significant increase in the amount of UV reaching the eye. Analysis of epidemiologic data in this study demonstrated also that sunglasses provide a

---

[20] Doheny, Kathleen, "More People—Even Kids—Need to Wear Sunglasses," WebMD. https://www.webmd.com/eye-health/news/20120517/more-people-even-kids-need-to-wear-sunglasses

[21] Tierney, Emily and C. William Hanke, "The Eyelids: Highly Susceptible to Skin Cancer," Skin Cancer Foundation. http://www.skincancer.org/prevention/sun-protection/for-your-eyes/the-eyelids-highly-susceptible-to-skin-cancer

photoprotective effect against both cataracts and periorbital (the area surrounding the eye) basal cell carcinoma."[22]

Sunglasses can prevent wind, sun and other objects from getting into your eye and causing damage, particularly the wraparound style with UV-protective side shields. Dry eye issues can be lessened by wearing sunglasses for the above reasons.[23]

Another benefit of wearing sunglasses is for those who experience cluster headaches, frequently occurring headaches or migraines. For some, bright sunlight can be a trigger, and wearing sunglasses can help reduce both the intensity and the frequency of these occurrences.[24]

As stated earlier, unshaded eyes exposed to sunlight can help serotonin and melatonin hormone levels. Dr. Neil Nedley recommends 30 minutes a day.[25] Gradually increase your time without sunglasses to get your eyes used to bright light if you are not accustomed to it. Never look directly into the sun.

Truly a blessing from God, the health benefits of sunlight are many. Proper clothing choices can help prevent damage from sun "worship."

"But unto you who revere and worshipfully fear My name shall the Sun of Righteousness arise

---

[22] Ibid.
[23] Hargrave Eye Center, "Health Benefits of Sunglasses," SlideShare. https://www.slideshare.net/hargraveeyecenter/health-benefits-of-sunglasses
[24] Artisan Optics, "The Health Benefits of Wearing Sunglasses," Artisan Optics. http://www.artisanoptics.com/artisan/blogs/jill_a__kronberg__od/e_993/The_Eyecare_Corner/2017/3/TheHealthBenefitsofWearingSunglasses.htm
[25] Nedley, 88.

with healing in His wings and His beams."
Malachi 4:2, AMPC

CHAPTER TWO

Keep Cool with Proper Clothing

The Second Commandment

"You shall not make for yourself a carved image—any likeness of anything that is in heaven above, or that is in the earth beneath, or that is in the water under the earth; you shall not bow down to them nor serve them. For I, the LORD your God, am a jealous God, visiting the iniquity of the fathers upon the children to the third and fourth generations of those who hate Me, but showing mercy to thousands, to those who love Me and keep My commandments."
Exodus 20: 4–6, NKJV

Principle

Keep cool with proper clothing, not by imitating fashion "idols."

In Genesis 3:21, we are told "for Adam also and for his wife the Lord God made long coats (tunics) of skins and clothed them" (AMPC). Our caring, merciful God provided not only an object lesson of the sacrifice of the cross of Christ but also the perfect outfit for their needs. "In humility and inexpressible sadness Adam and Eve left the lovely garden wherein they had been so happy until they disobeyed the command of God. The atmosphere was changed. It was no longer unvarying as before the transgression. God clothed them with coats of skins to protect them from the sense of chilliness and then of heat to which they were exposed."[26]

Adam and Eve, not fully understanding their needs, had unsuccessfully attempted to properly clothe themselves. "Then the eyes of them both were opened, and they knew that they were naked; and they sewed fig leaves together and made themselves apronlike girdles" (Genesis 3:7, AMPC). The outfits they sewed were inadequate for their health and comfort. Similarly, current warm weather fashions often have minimal fabric and maximum skin exposure, conveying the idea that keeping the body cool requires little coverage. Our physiology, however, teaches us a different perspective.

"Just as the body must be protected from becoming too cold, it must also be protected from excessively high temperatures. Most heat loss occurs through the skin via radiation or evaporation. When body temperature increases above what is desirable, the blood vessels serving the skin dilate and capillary beds in the skin become flushed with warm blood. As a result, heat radiates from the skin surface. However, if the external environment is as hot as or hotter that the body, heat cannot be lost by radiation, and the only means of getting rid of excess heat is by evaporation of perspiration off the skin surface. This is an efficient means of body-heat loss as long as the air is dry. If it is humid, evaporation occurs at a much slower rate. In such cases, our heat-liberating mechanisms don't work well, and we feel miserable and irritable."[27]

---

[26] White, E. G. (1947). *The Story of Redemption*. Hagerstown, MD: Review and Herald Publishing Association, 46.

[27] Marieb, Elaine (2006) *Essentials of Human Anatomy & Physiology*, eighth edition. San Francisco, CA: Pearson Benjamin Cummings, 488, 490.

It can indeed be a challenge to be comfortable and healthy in hot weather. The list below is advice from the late Dr. Agatha Thrash, which she titled, "How to Keep Cool."[28]

A. Dress against the heat.

- Protect the skin from direct rays of the sun by loose clothing of cotton material that fully covers the arms and the legs. In countries where the weather is very hot, clothing is loose fitting and covers the body well.
- Choose light colors which reflect the heat and thus keep the body cool.
- Wearing long sleeves both summer and winter prevents the "alarm reaction" of the adrenals that causes a vigorous adjustment in the nervous system and the sensation of extreme overheating if even a light sleeve is worn. The reaction is paradoxically characterized by an intolerance to covering the arms. It is an adaptation response of the nervous system to the stress of chilling.

B. Keep the head cool while in the sun by wearing a hat, avoiding the midday sun when possible, and by drinking plenty of water to promote free sweating.

C. Eat lighter foods, emphasizing fresh fruits and vegetables. Heavy or sweet foods, fatty foods, or high protein foods cause much heat production.

---

[28] Thrash, Agatha, "Clothing," Uchee Pines. https://www.ucheepines.org/clothing/

D. Water. Perspiration can be promoted by drinking much water, and the natural temperature controls of the body, the skin and lungs, can be much more efficient if there is plenty of water.[29]

Women experiencing hot flashes or night sweats in perimenopause and menopause have additional challenges regarding clothing. They can benefit by learning to dress in a way that does not exacerbate or intensify hot flashes. An understanding of physiology can assist women in dressing appropriately for this condition.

"A hot flash is a quick feeling of heat and sometimes a red, flushed face and sweating. The exact cause of hot flashes is not known, but they may be related to changes in circulation. Hot flashes happen when the blood vessels near the skin's surface dilate to cool, making you break out in a sweat."[30] "Some researchers suggest it might have to do with mixed signals from the hypothalamus, a region in the brain that regulates body temperature and sex hormones. The hypothalamus may be reacting to decreasing levels of estrogen, and this may explain why hot flashes cease when estrogen replacement is given."[31]

Prior to discussing clothing principles for women with hot flashes, a few important points about estrogen replacement therapy and alternatives seems appropriate. "Women who took either combined hormone therapy or estrogen alone had an increased risk

---

[29] Ibid.

[30] WebMD, "What Are Hot Flashes?," WebMD. https://www.webmd.com/menopause/guide/menopause-hot-flashes

[31] Weil, Andrew, "Menopause Symptoms and Treatments," Dr. Weil. https://www.drweil.com/health-wellness/health-centers/women/menopause-symptoms-and-treatments/

of stroke, blood clots, and heart attack."[32] In addition, "risk of breast cancer from estrogen alone or estrogen combined with progesterone is also increased."[33] Alternatives to HRT include bioidentical hormones and herbs, food and supplements which can aid hormone balance.

Dr. Andrew Weil advises women to "try the following natural remedies and menopause treatments, including herbs:"[34]

Soy foods. The isoflavones in soy foods help balance hormone levels and have some estrogenic activity. There is ongoing research about the safety and efficacy of isolated soy isoflavone supplements. While the initial results look promising, we currently recommend using natural soy foods rather than supplements. Choose from tofu, soy milk, roasted soy nuts or tempeh.

Flaxseed. Substances called lignins in flaxseed are important modulators of hormone metabolism. Grind flaxseed daily in a coffee grinder at home and use 1 to 2 tablespoons a day.

---

[32] National Cancer Institute, "Menopausal Hormone Therapy and Cancer," NIH https://www.cancer.gov/about-cancer/causes-prevention/risk/hormones/mht-fact-sheet
[33] Weil, Andrew, "How Dangerous is Hormone Replacement Therapy?," Dr. Weil https://www.drweil.com/health-wellness/health-centers/women/how-dangerous-is-hormone-replacement-therapy/
[34] Weil, Andrew, "Menopause Symptoms and Treatments, Dr. Weil. https://www.drweil.com/health-wellness/health-centers/women/menopause-symptoms-and-treatments/

Dong quai. Dong quai (*Angelica sinensis*) is known both in China and the West for its ability to support and maintain the natural balance of female hormones. It does not have estrogenic activity.

This is one of the herbs for menopause that should not be taken if a woman is experiencing heavy bleeding.

Black cohosh (*Cumicifuga racemosa*). One of the best-studied traditional herbs for menopause, black cohosh is used to help alleviate some symptoms of menopause, and is considered an effective hot flash remedy. Black cohosh seems to work by supporting and maintaining hormonal levels, which may lessen the severity of hot flashes. Many women report that the herb works well but it isn't effective for everyone. While any therapy that influences hormonal actions should be a concern, black cohosh does not appear to have estrogenic activity and thus may be safe for women with a personal or family history of breast cancer.

Vitamin E. A daily dose of 400 IUs of natural vitamin E (as mixed tocopherols and tocotrienols) can help alleviate symptoms of hot flashes in some menopausal women.

B vitamins. This group of water-soluble vitamins may help women deal with the stress of menopausal symptoms.

Evening primrose oil or black currant oil. These are sources of gamma-linolenic acid (GLA), an essential fatty acid that can help influence prostaglandin synthesis and help moderate menopausal symptoms.

Another natural option is deep breathing. "A deep breathing exercise will often stop a hot flash in a few seconds. Simply breathe in deeply through the nose and out through the mouth, repeatedly, until the flash stops."[35] This can be particularly helpful if the woman breathes deeply of cool air, such as standing in outdoor winter air, inhaling near an open kitchen freezer or using a small hand-held fan to the face.

Due to the sudden nature of hot flashes, a practical approach for clothing year-round is to wear layers which can be easily removed when a hot flash occurs. The use of scarves, blazers and cardigans are better options than pullover and turtleneck sweaters for ease of removal, as well as appropriate for professional dress codes.

Fabric is also important to consider with hot flashes, to facilitate moisture evaporation and skin cooling. "Make sure to wear fabrics that are breathable and allow air to flow in and out. Cotton is usually the go-to option, and is seen as a more affordable fabric. A nice cotton shirt, paired with some looser khaki pants, is the perfect weekend outfit to keep you cool, even during the summer months. Linen is also a good fabric option and it dresses up nicely."[36] For sleepwear when experiencing night sweats, there are companies which market moisture-wicking nightgowns and pajama sets. Cotton bed linens are often beneficial, as well.[37] For those with a more sizeable budget, Charla Blacker, MD, an obstetrician-gynecologist at Henry Ford

---

[35] Thrash, Agatha, "Menopause Assistance," Uchee Pines. https://www.ucheepines.org/menopause-assistance/

[36] 34 Menopause Symptoms, "How to Dress for Hot Flashes," 34 Menopause Symptoms.
 https://www.34-menopause-symptoms.com/hot-flashes/articles/how-to-dress-for-hot-flashes.htm

[37] Durning, Marijke Vroomen and Erica Roth, "Understanding and Dealing with Hot Flashes," Healthline.
https://www.healthline.com/health/menopause/understanding-hot-flashes

Hospital in Detroit, "suggests sleeping in light, breathable silk pajamas or on cool silk sheets to help turn down the heat."[38]

Preventing hot flashes through understanding triggers is extremely helpful. "They can be triggered by tight clothing, stress, or consuming alcohol, caffeine, and spicy foods."[39] Other triggers include a hot environment and cigarette smoking or second-hand smoke.

Not only is tight-fitting clothing a health issue for circulation, which will be discussed in a subsequent chapter, but also for hot flashes. "Experiencing a hot flash when wearing something tight-fitting and stuffy can be a nightmare. Lots of beautiful clothing is made to be loose fitting, and utilizing it can help you to better handle hot flashes. Flowing skirts, loose tops, and gaucho pants can all help you to keep cool. Looser fitting clothes are also less likely to show sweat."[40]

When choosing exercise clothing, women with hot flashes can benefit from lightweight, breathable fabrics designed for exercise. Dr. Agatha Thrash recommended "a woman obtain three to five

---

[38] Bowers, Elizabeth Shimer, "7 Surprising Benefits of Silk," Everyday Health.
https://www.everydayhealth.com/skin-and-beauty-pictures/surprising-benefits-of-silk.aspx#02

[39] Durning, Marijke Vroomen and Erica Roth, "Understanding and Dealing with Hot Flashes," Healthline.
https://www.healthline.com/health/menopause/understanding-hot-flashes

[40] 34 Menopause Symptoms, "How to Dress for Hot Flashes," 34 Menopause Symptoms.
https://www.34-menopause-symptoms.com/hot-flashes/articles/how-to-dress-for-hot-flashes.htm

hours of outdoor labor daily to stimulate the ovaries and other endocrine glands."[41] For women who cannot exercise as long a time, there are still benefits from exercise. "Though frequent workouts haven't been proven as a means of reducing menopausal symptoms, they can ease the transition by helping to relieve stress and enhance your overall quality of life. Regular exercise is also an excellent way to stave off weight gain and loss of muscle mass, which are two frequent symptoms of menopause."[42]

Albeit challenging, keeping cool in warm weather and during hot flashes can be greatly aided by proper clothing and a healthy lifestyle. God's timeless principles can benefit every generation.

> *"Turn away my eyes from beholding vanity (idols and idolatry); and restore me to vigorous life and health in Your ways."*
> *Psalm 119:37, AMPC*

---

[41] Thrash, Agatha, "Menopause Assistance," Uchee Pines. https://www.ucheepines.org/menopause-assistance/

[42] Cappelloni, Lisa, "The Best Activities to Do During Menopause," Healthline. https://www.healthline.com/health-slideshow/ten-best-menopause-activities#2

CHAPTER THREE

Keep Warm with Adequate Clothing

The Third Commandment

"You shall not take the name of the LORD *your God in vain, for the* LORD *will not hold him guiltless who takes His name in vain."*
Exodus 20: 7, NKJV

Principle

Keeping warm with adequate clothing honors the name of the Lord, Jehovah Jireh, "The Lord Who Provides."

Our loving Lord knows we need to be warm enough in cold weather, and cool enough in hot weather, for our health and happiness. He created us with perceptions of being heated or chilled for our body's protection.

Our caring Divine Designer has fashioned our bodies to work on the principle of homeostasis. Homeostasis is defined as "a relative constancy in the internal environment of the body, naturally maintained by adaptive responses that promote healthy survival. Various sensing, feedback, and control mechanisms function to effect this steady state. Some of the key control mechanisms are the reticular formation in the brainstem and the endocrine glands. Some of the functions controlled by homeostatic mechanisms are heartbeat, hematopoiesis, blood pressure, body temperature, electrolytic balance, respiration, and glandular secretion."[43]

Our internal body temperature is carefully maintained by several of the systems of our bodies, in order to ensure an internal reading of 98.6° F (37.0° C), when in health.

"When the environmental temperature is cold (or the temperature of circulating blood falls), body heat must be conserved (increased). Short-term mean of accomplishing this are vasoconstriction of blood vessels of the skin and shivering.

"When the skin vasculature constricts, the skin is temporarily bypassed by the blood, and blood is rerouted to the deeper, more vital, body organs. When this happens, the temperature of the exposed skin drops to that of the external environment. . . .

"When the *core* body temperature (the temperature of the deep organs) drops to the point beyond which simple constriction of skin capillaries can handle the situation, shivering begins. Shivering, involuntary shudderlike contractions of the voluntary muscles, is very effective in increasing the body temperature, because skeletal muscle activity produces large amounts of heat. . . ."[44]

"Animal experiments are very clear in showing the profound changes in various organs due to the stress of chilling. To the general stressful factors of modern life must be added the stress of improper clothing."[45]

"It is impossible to have the best of health if the extremities are habitually cold. The unequal circulation which results from

---

[43] Medical Dictionary, "Homeostasis," The Free Dictionary. http://medical-dictionary.thefreedictionary.com/homeostasis

[44] Marieb, Elaine (2006) *Essentials of Human Anatomy & Physiology*, eighth edition. San Francisco, CA: Pearson Benjamin Cummings, 488.

[45] Thrash, Agatha, "Healthful Body Temperature," Uchee Pines. http://www.ucheepines.org/healthful-body-temperature/

clothing the trunk more warmly than the extremities allows toxic materials to build up both in the anemic extremities and in the congested viscera. Blood tends to pool in any area of inflammation. In the head the excess blood produces headaches, in the chest it produces coughs, in the intestinal tract various types of discomfort, and in the kidneys inefficient cleaning of the blood. The nervous system responds to messages from chilled areas with an alarm reaction."[46] "There are some who are so sensitive to chilling of the extremities that they get high blood pressure if the feet are even slightly chilled."[47]

The late Dr. Agatha Thrash told me that "the worst thing you can do to your health is to become chilled."[48] She explained to me that the best test for ensuring the warmth, and therefore the circulation, of the extremities is to touch your forehead, and then touch your arms and legs, to see if they are as warm as the forehead. If they are not, then a layer of clothing is needed.

The Holy Bible also teaches us the importance of wearing layers in cold conditions. We are told that this is one way the wise, virtuous woman described in Proverbs, chapter 31, dressed herself and her family to protect them from the cold. "She is not afraid of the snow for her household: for all her household [are] clothed with scarlet" [Margin: double garments] (Proverbs 31:21, KJV).

"Much of the feebleness which is suffered by women is the result of improper clothing of the extremities. Congestion of the pelvic organs can lead to cervicitis, dysmenorrhea, cervical polyps,

---

[46] Thrash, Agatha, "Clothing," Uchee Pines. http://www.ucheepines.org/clothing/

[47] Thrash, Agatha, "My Experience with Dress Reform," Uchee Pines. http://www.ucheepines.org/my-experience-with-dress-reform/

[48] Thrash, Agatha. Personal communication, July, 1992.

and malpositions of the uterus. In pregnancy the placenta may not get a sufficient circulation of the blood. As a result of a sluggish exchange of blood, the development of the fetus may be retarded. Vitality is expended unnecessarily to supply the want of sufficient clothing. Usually proper dress demands warm underclothing."[49]

"The susceptibility to viral infections is greatly increased if the extremities are not kept warmly clad at all times. . . . We have fixed macrophages in the skin which are important in combating disease. If the blood can be flooded past these important structures, they assist in protecting against infection, particularly upper respiratory tract infections. Many diseases that have long been elusive as to cause are now being considered as virus diseases. These include such diseases as cancer, arthritis, ulcerative colitis, etc. We may lower the body's resistance to these types of disease by improperly clothing the extremities."[50]

"[An] evil which custom fosters is the unequal distribution of the clothing, so that while some parts of the body have more than is required, others are insufficiently clad. The feet and limbs, being remote from the vital organs, should be especially guarded from cold by abundant clothing. It is impossible to have health when the extremities are habitually cold; for if there is too little blood in them there will be too much in other portions of the body. Perfect health requires a perfect circulation; but this cannot be had while three or four times as much clothing is worn upon the body, where the vital organs are situated, as upon the feet and limbs."[51]

---

[49] Thrash, Agatha, "Clothing," Uchee Pines. http://www.ucheepines.org/clothing/
[50] Ibid.
[51] White, E. G. (1905). *The Ministry of Healing*. Mountain View, CA: Pacific Press Publishing Association, 293.

When "the extremities are chilled, and the heart has thrown upon it double labor, to force the blood into these chilled extremities, and when the blood has performed its circuit through the body, and returned to the heart, it is not the same vigorous warm current which left it. It has been chilled in its passage through the limbs. The heart, weakened by too great labor, and poor circulation of poor blood, is then compelled to still greater exertion, to throw the blood to the extremities which are never as healthfully warm as other parts of the body. The heart fails in its efforts, and the limbs become habitually cold; and the blood, which is chilled away from the extremities, is thrown back upon the lungs and brain, and inflammation and congestion of the lungs or the brain is the result."[52]

"Warm underclothing and footgear are the secret to keeping warm in cool weather. Increasing the number of layers of a substantial fabric until the effects of the weather are no longer felt will be effective in bringing warmth to the skin. This principle is poorly understood by most women, who do not have any idea why their feet are habitually cold. The feet and legs are essentially naked. Gossamer [light, thin] hosiery and thin-soled shoes are scanty protection against morbid chilling. Hot footbaths are necessary to bring the temperature up to normal levels.

"What is required is several layers of quite warm fabric, perhaps bulky, covered by substantial shoes [or boots] and warm basic garments (dress, pants). The underclothing and hose should be warm enough to give adequate protection against chilling, almost

---

[52] White, E. G. (1958). *Selected Messages Book 2*. Washington, D.C.: Review and Herald Publishing Association. 470.

unaided by top clothing. Then the top and overclothes are not the major protectors from chilling."[53]

Several years ago, I learned by personal experience the great value of dressing with regard to maintaining the warmth of the arms and legs with adequate layers of carefully planned clothing. At that time, I had been diagnosed with fibromyalgia. The searing pain in all my extremities was disabling. I searched and tried various traditional and alternative medical treatments without success. Our wonderful Divine Physician guided me to the perfect solution — my clothing! As long as I kept all my extremities warm, including care in air conditioning during the summer, I was able to function and find pain relief. If I neglected to wear clothing which kept my extremities warm enough, the knife-like pain would return.

Our loving Heavenly Father wants us to be warm, healthy and happy. He created our wonderful bodies with the ability to sense chilliness to encourage us to adequately clothe ourselves, in order to maintain our circulation and help our resistance to disease.

"Now this is what the LORD Almighty says: 'Give careful thought to your ways. You have planted much, but harvested little. You eat, but never have enough. You drink, but never have your fill. You put on clothes, but are not warm. You earn wages, only to put them in a purse with holes.'"
Haggai 1:5, 6. NIV

---

[53] Thrash, Agatha, "Healthful Body Temperature," Uchee Pines. http://www.ucheepines.org/healthful-body-temperature/

CHAPTER FOUR

Dressing for Healthful Circulation

The Fourth Commandment

"Remember the Sabbath day, to keep it holy. Six days you shall labor and do all your work, but the seventh day is the Sabbath of the LORD your God. In it you shall do no work: you, nor your son, nor your daughter, nor your male servant, nor your female servant, nor your cattle, nor your stranger who is within your gates. For in six days the LORD made the heavens and the earth, the sea, and all that is in them, and rested the seventh day. Therefore the LORD blessed the Sabbath day and hallowed it."
Exodus 20: 8 – 11, NKJV

Principle

Healthful clothing allows our circulation to flow "wholly," blessing every cell.

Now that we have learned how important clothing is for our wonderful bodies' temperature control, we may want to exclaim with the psalmist David, "I will praise You, for I am fearfully and wonderfully made; marvelous are Your works, and that my soul knows very well" (Psalm 139:14, NKJV). Our wise Creator also wants to bless us by being informed how to have carefree compression from our clothing, so that we can have optimal circulation of our blood and lymphatic fluid. Circulation which flows "wholly" contributes to the healthy function of our valued organs, including our lovely skin, by reaching every cell in our body.

The Holy Scriptures tell us that "the life of the flesh is in the blood" (Leviticus 17:11, KJV). All our precious cells are nourished by nutrients, and protected by leukocytes and immune factors, which circulate in our blood and lymphatic circulation. Waste products and toxins are removed from our cells by our blood-filled veins and our lymphatic vessels. This is why it is of the utmost importance that our lifestyle habits, including how we dress, benefit our circulation of blood and lymph fluid rather than hindering its free course. "Perfect health depends upon perfect circulation."[54]

In her book *Fashion Victim*, Michelle Lee also quotes Ellen G. White, who she recognizes as a Rational Dress supporter: "A bad circulation leaves the blood to become impure, and induces congestion of the brain and lungs, and causes diseases of the head, the heart, the liver, and the lungs. The fashionable style of woman's dress is one of the greatest causes of all these terrible diseases."[55]

It is important that our pretty clothes fit us well, yet do not cause us harm from excess pressure or restriction of natural, graceful movement. "Any bands that impede the circulation or leave a mark on the skin or prevent entirely free motion of an extremity are improper."[56]

"Of late years the dangers resulting from compression of the waist have been so fully discussed that few can be ignorant in regard to them; yet so great is the power of fashion that the evil continues.

---

[54] White, E. G. (1952). *My Life Today*. Washington, D.C.: Review and Herald Publishing Association, 145.

[55] Lee, Michelle (2003) *Fashion Victim*. New York: Broadway Books, 216. [Originally published by E.G. White (August 1, 1868) "The Dress Reform," *The Health Reformer*.]

[56] Thrash, Agatha, "Clothing," Uchee Pines. http://www.ucheepines.org/clothing/

By this practice, women and young girls are doing themselves untold harm. It is essential to health that the chest have room to expand to its fullest extent in order that the lungs may be enabled to take full inspiration. When the lungs are restricted, the quantity of oxygen received into them is lessened. The blood is not properly vitalized, and the waste, poisonous matter which should be thrown off through the lungs is retained. In addition to this the circulation is hindered, and the internal organs are so cramped and crowded out of place that they cannot perform their work properly.

"Tight lacing does not improve the form. One of the chief elements in physical beauty is symmetry, the harmonious proportion of parts. And the correct model for physical development is to be found, not in the figures displayed by French modistes, but in the human form as developed according to the laws of God in nature. God is the author of all beauty, and only as we conform to His ideal shall we approach the standard of true beauty."[57]

Our lovely Savior Jesus wants us to be lovely, too. His ideal of beauty is so much higher and lovelier than what is considered beautiful in our culture. "For as the heavens are higher than the earth, so are My ways higher than your ways, and My thoughts than your thoughts" (Isaiah 55:9). Yet in an effort to portray a contemporary ideal feminine figure, some women are hurting their tender organs.

In an article entitled, "Spanx and Other Shapewear are Literally Squeezing Your Organs," it is reported that "shapewear couldn't do its job if it wasn't tight. Unfortunately, this leaves your stomach, intestine and colon compressed, which Dr. [John] Kuemmerle [a gastroenterologist] says can worsen acid reflux and heartburn. Restrictive clothing can also provoke erosive

---

[57] White, E. G. (1905). *The Ministry of Healing*. Mountain View, CA: Pacific Press Publishing Association, 292.

esophagitis." It also "can lead to unpleasant symptoms like abdominal discomfort, bloating and gas.

"Another hallmark of shapewear? Shallow breath. When you inhale, your diaphragm expands and your abdomen flares out, Dr. Erickson [a chiropractor] says, but shapewear restricts this movement and decreases the excursion in respiration.

"Sitting in shapewear can lead to a reversible condition called meralgia paresthetica, which is when the peripheral nerve in your thigh is compressed. This leads to tingling, numbness and pain in your legs, all of which can come and go *or* become constant. "It's like putting these giant rubber bands around your upper thighs and tightening them when you sit," Dr. Erickson says. (She's also seen this condition in those who wear too-tight pantyhose and pants.)

"This rubber band effect can also decrease your circulation and lead to blood clots. When you sit in shapewear, Dr. Erickson explains that those genetically prone to varicosities can develop varicose veins and lymph congestion, which manifests as swollen ankles.

"Shapewear is occlusive, meaning it traps moisture and anything else under it, which predisposes shapewear wearers to both yeast and bacterial infections. Dr. [Maryann] Mikhail [a dermatologist] says that the most common infection she sees is folliculitis, since bacteria often gets trapped among hair follicles."[58]

"Tight garments on the lower abdominal region and the upper thigh can cause a condition called meralgia paresthetica, irritation of the nerves in the front and outer aspects of the thigh,"

---

[58] Adams, Rebecca, "Spanx and Other Shapewear Are Literally Squeezing Your Organs," Huffington Post. http://www.huffingtonpost.com/2014/01/20/spanx-shapewear_n_4616907.html

says Orly Avitzur, M.D., a neurologist and medical adviser to Consumer Reports who practices in Carmel, N.Y.

"We've known about this for many years and used to see it in women who wore girdles. Now we see it in other compression garments, which have become quite a common fashion accessory. So we're seeing more and more of that in this generation of women who are trying to look sleek in their clothing." Symptoms include burning, pain, tingling in the thigh area and hypersensitivity to the touch, according to Dr. Avitzur.[59]

Edward R. Laskowski, M.D. acknowledges that "although you may appear thinner when you wear a girdle, the girdle doesn't strengthen or tone your abdominal muscles. Girdles just temporarily compress and redistribute fat and skin around the abdomen. When it comes to a flat stomach, diet and exercise—not undergarments—are what count."

"Dietary changes and aerobic exercise can help you shed unwanted pounds, including those around your middle. Although it takes aerobic activity to burn fat, core exercises can strengthen and tone the underlying muscles.

"Core exercises include abdominal crunches, leg lifts, plank poses and bridge poses."[60]

---

[59] Clayton, Jamie Dalessio, "5 Ways Clothing Can Make You Sick," Everyday Health.
http://www.everydayhealth.com/pain-management-pictures/ways-clothing-can-make-you-sick.aspx#06

[60] Laskowski, Edward, "Can wearing a girdle help tighten stomach muscles?" Mayo Clinic Healthy-Lifestyle.
http://www.mayoclinic.org/healthy-lifestyle/fitness/expert-answers/flat-stomach/faq-20058288

Several years ago I was asked to share a short talk on weight control with a sweet audience of teenage girls. My abbreviated list of information was based on ageless principles of how to healthfully reduce caloric intake, which can help reduce abdominal girth and adipose tissue. These are the three weight loss tips I shared:

1. Drink only water or herb teas between meals

2. Do not eat between meals

3. Eat only unrefined foods that contain fiber (i.e. whole plant foods)

In order to reduce the need for a girdle because of abdominal bloating, determining one's food allergies and sensitivities can be helpful. An allergist or other health care professional can help determine the foods to which you are allergic. An elimination diet can help, in addition, to provide a means of knowing to which foods you react, and are therefore sensitive to without a true immune allergic reaction. A valuable resource is the book *Food Allergies Made Simple*, by Phylis Austin, Agatha Thrash, MD and Calvin Thrash, MD.

Tight pants can contribute to other uncomfortable, even hurtful digestive issues. "Pressure on the stomach, known as intragastric pressure or intra-abdominal pressure, can trigger acid reflux—pushing stomach acid back up through the lower esophageal junction, where the esophagus and the stomach meet, causing heartburn.

"Acid reflux is common, and not just for older adults, according to Dr. Koufman, who says about 37 percent of the 20 to 30-year-old age group gets it. Even someone who isn't prone to acid reflux can develop reflux if they wear a tight article of clothing often over a two-week period, she says. Snug-fitting corset-style shirts can have a similar effect, says Koufman."[61]

"Tight corsets, which compress the lungs, the stomach, and other internal organs, and induce curvature of the spine and an almost countless train of diseases."[62] "My sisters, there is need of a dress reform among us. There are many errors in the present style of female dress. It is injurious to health, and, therefore, sin for females to wear tight corsets . . . or to compress the waist. These have a depressing influence upon the heart, liver, and lungs. The health of the entire system depends upon the healthy action of the respiratory organs. Thousands of females have ruined their constitutions, and brought upon themselves various diseases, in their efforts to make a healthy and natural form unhealthy and unnatural."[63]

Our health may also be affected by wearing pants that are just too tight for unimpaired circulation. "The way a woman wears her slacks might leave her prone to the breakdown of fatty tissue at the outside of the thighs, called lipoatrophia semicircularis, dermatologists say. "Persistent mechanical pressure" exerted by "strangling folds" of too-tight trousers can impair circulation and set the stage for this condition, especially in women who sit for long periods, according to a study from Chile's Universidad Andres Bello in the June 2007 Journal of Dermatology."[64]

---

[61] Clayton, Jamie Dalessio, "5 Ways Clothing Can Make You Sick," Everyday Health. http://www.everydayhealth.com/pain-management-pictures/ways-clothing-can-make-you-sick.aspx#06

[62] White, E. G. (1923). *Counsels on Health*. Mountain View, CA: Pacific Press Publishing Association, 599.

[63] White, E. G. (1958). *Selected Messages Book 2*. Washington, D.C.: Review and Herald Publishing Association, 473.

[64] Allen, Jane E. "Wardrobe Woes: Hidden Health Hazards of Clothing," ABC News Medical Unit.

As rivers which flow unhindered bless the neighboring trees with life-giving water during a drought, so our blood and lymphatic fluid will bless our organs and cells when we wear clothing which does not hinder its free circulation.

"If you diligently heed the voice of the Lord your God and do what is right in His sight, give ear to His commandments and keep all His statutes, I will put none of the diseases on you which I have brought on the Egyptians. For I am the Lord who heals you."
Exodus 15:26, NKJV

---

http://abcnews.go.com/Health/wardrobe-woes-hidden-health-hazards-clothing/story?id=15761031

CHAPTER FIVE

Honor Your Feminine Organs

The Fifth Commandment

*"Honor your father and your mother,
as the* LORD *your God has commanded you,
that your days may be long, and that it may be well with you in
the land which the* LORD *your God is giving you."*
Deuteronomy 5: 16, NKJV

Principle

Honor your inherited feminine organs with healthy garments.

In the Garden of Eden, "God Himself gave Adam a companion... Eve was created from a rib taken from the side of Adam, signifying that she was not to control him as the head, nor to be trampled under his feet as an inferior, but to stand by his side as an equal, to be loved and protected by him. A part of man, bone of his bone, and flesh of his flesh, she was his second self; showing the close union and the affectionate attachment that should exist in this relation."[65]

---

[65] White, E. G. (1952). *The Adventist Home.* Hagerstown, MD: Review and Herald Publishing Association, 25.

Beautiful Eve was different, yet equal. These feminine differences in women's bodies underlie the special needs for women's clothing to support and not hinder health.

There are some who are concerned that our bras may affect the health of our breasts. Michelle Lee sites medical anthropologists Sydney and Soma Singer, authors of the book *Dressed to Kill*, who "blamed bras for causing breast cancer, claiming that compression constricts the lymphatic system, the body's natural means of ridding itself of toxins."[66] I have heard the testimony of three women who share not only the diagnosis of breast cancer, but all three state that their malignant tumors grew in the exact place where the underwire of their bras had rubbed and caused irritation. I do not claim this as a definitive cause-and-effect relationship, but one certainly would wonder if it is a contributing factor.

"If your bra leaves red marks that last for more than 20 minutes once you have removed it, it's too tight. If your shoulder straps leave marks on the top of your shoulders or the straps are digging in, your bra isn't doing its job correctly. Underwire bras can put pressure on the tissue beneath, restricting lymphatic circulation. Minimize how many hours a day you wear a bra or other restrictive garment. Find a bra with wider, softer shoulder straps if you are large-breasted, and avoid underwire bras."[67]

Mary Brace Denka, a massage therapist who works with athletic clients, states, "Sports bras can make the torso rigid and I

---

[66] Lee, Michelle (2003) *Fashion Victim*. New York: Broadway Books, 225.

[67] Groulx, Julie, "What Restricts Your Lympahatic Circulation?" MammAlive. The Healthy Breast Program. http://mammalive.net/mind-body-practices/restricts-lymphatic-circulation/

have seen them causing the intercostals to tense up, reducing the ability to breathe deeply."[68]

As much as we like to be comfortable and warm, there are times, however, when too much warmth is unhealthy. "If the breasts are more warmly clothed than the extremities, the resulting increased temperature makes them susceptible to various diseases, from inability to nurse one's infant, to cystic disease and various tumors. The normal temperature of the breast is several degrees below that of the surrounding skin. Mammary thermograms show an increased breast temperature in breast cancer and many benign lesions."[69] "Overheating the breasts by padding or by wearing many layers of clothing on the trunk and few or none on the extremities leads to congestion of the breasts, and can keep the temperature of these delicate organs several degrees above normal. It is suggested that just as overheating the testes can lead to cancer in these organs, so overheating the breasts can lead to cancer and other breast diseases."[70]

Breast augmentation is opted by some women, rather than wearing heavily-padded bras. Several potential health risks, although low in percentage of occurrence, have been noted by reconstructive surgeon Clara Lee, MD. These include risk of post-operative infection, leakage of silicone or saline-filled implants,

---

[68] Denka, Mary Brace, Personal Communication, September 13, 2017.

[69] Thrash, Agatha, "Clothing," Uchee Pines. http://www.ucheepines.org/clothing/

[70] Thrash, Agatha, "Dress for Our Day," Uchee Pines. http://www.ucheepines.org/dress-for-our-day/

capsular contracture of scar tissue, and a slow-growing cancer, anaplastic large cell lymphoma (ALCL).[71]

Clothing can also affect a woman's delicate reproductive organs. Wearing tight garments can have adverse effects upon pelvic organs. "Research carried out by Professor John Dickinson of the Wolfson Institute of Preventive Medicine and published in the British Journal of Obstetrics and Gynaecology links tight clothing to endometriosis, a gynaecological medical condition that can cause infertility in women.

"The study titled *Could tight garments cause endometriosis?* says tight clothes may provide the force required to drive endometrial cells from the womb to accumulate in the ovaries.

"Professor Dickinson points out that the garments a woman wears during her menstrual days could be important.

"'If the garments are so tight-fitting as to produce even a small sustained rise of intra-abdominal solid tissue pressure, retrograde menstruation is likely to occur when the garments are removed and when the salpingo-uterine junction is relaxed between uterine contractions,' he notes."[72]

During menstruation, most Western women wear tampons and/or sanitary pads. These are manufactured of different quality materials, and may potentially affect health, as well.

---

[71] Birch, Jenna, "These Are the Risks of Breast Implants, According to a Surgeon," Health. http://www.health.com/mind-body/breast-implants-cancer-other-risks

[72] Wakhisi, Sylvia, "Why Tight Clothing Exposes You to a Serious Number of Health Risks," Evewoman. http://www.standardmedia.co.ke/evewoman/m/article/2000120472/why-tight-clothing-exposes-you-to-a-number-of-serious-health-risks

"Plasticizing chemicals like BPA and BPS disrupt embryonic development and are linked to heart disease and cancer. Phthalates—which give paper tampon applicators that smooth feel and finish—are known to dysregulate gene expression, and DEHP may lead to multiple organ damage. Besides crude oil plastics, conventional sanitary pads can also contain a myriad of other potentially hazardous ingredients, such as odor neutralizers and fragrances. Synthetics and plastic also restrict the free flow of air and can trap heat and dampness, potentially promoting the growth of yeast and bacteria in your vaginal area."[73] The labia and vaginal area is highly vascular, making it easier for harmful chemicals to enter the body.

Natural cotton and organic menstrual products are opted by some women, in order to avoid potential risks. Here is one woman's experience:

"I've struggled with heavy cycles for seven years, and have had two blood transfusions and 2 years of iron infusions for anemia as a result. I started using holistic measures (i.e. diet and lifestyle) to determine the root cause. I stopped eating meat, greatly reduced dairy and increased exercise. I also maintained a better sleep regimen and increased sunlight, in addition to taking progesterone cream. While these all helped to reduce the bleeding, my cycles were still heavy. Within the last three months I've started using organic tampons and natural cotton pads. It's made a significant difference in addition to the other holistic measures and I can now see my cycle normalizing."[74]

---

[73] Mercola, Joseph, "Women Beware: Most Feminine Hygiene Products Contain Toxic Ingredients," Dr. Mercola. https://articles.mercola.com/sites/articles/archive/2013/05/22/feminine-hygiene-products.aspx

[74] Gary, Denetra. Personal Communication, October 13, 2017.

The choice of panties can also affect women's health. The fabric, fit, length of wear and shape all have an impact.

"Many doctors . . . advise going without underwear at night . . . and say it is inadvisable to wear panties 24 hours a day, to avoid vaginal infections.

"No underwear causes a whole host of other problems, particularly because clothing doesn't tend to have a liner," says Dr. Dardik. "For one, if you're wearing pants, the seam sits right in the vulval area and will constantly be rubbing the area," which can irritate sensitive tissue. Secondly, the natural moisture produced by the vagina has nowhere to go when you're not wearing underwear. "If you are wearing dresses or skirts, there's nothing there to absorb vaginal moisture," she adds. "Then you can become hot and sweaty down there, which, in itself, can irritate the skin."[75]

Cotton is often the recommended fabric for underwear. "'Wear loose, white cotton underwear; synthetic fabrics, as well as dyes, can be irritating,' advise Drs. Isabelle Labrie and Vincent Nadon, [of] the University of Ottawa.

"Many doctors advise wearing cotton underwear under pantyhose as well and to avoid nylon underwear and tight pantyhose, which cause increased perspiration and retention of heat and moisture. That creates a breeding ground for vaginal infections.

"All women secrete moisture and mucus from the membranes that line the vagina. It normally causes no irritation or inflammation, women's health advocates explain. And bacteria are natural to the vagina, as well.

---

[75] Schwartz, Sara, "8 Underwear Mistakes That Are Bad For Your Health," Huffington Post.

https://www.huffingtonpost.com/entry/8-underwear-mistakes-that-are-bad-for-your-health_us_5602b6dbe4b00310edf95264

"But when irritating cleansers are used, or feminine hygiene sprays and vaginal douches, irritation can result. The same is true for wearing underwear with fibers unsuited for good vaginal health."[76]

Another fabric for underwear reported to have health benefits is silk. "In the area of women's health, new Italian research shows that silk underwear may reduce itching and redness associated with recurrent vaginal yeast infections. Half of study participants wore briefs made from Dermasilk, and the other half wore cotton. After six months, 90 percent of the silk group had fewer symptoms, and recurrences were decreased by 50 percent. 'DermaSilk's antimicrobial properties and unique fiber weaving prevent it from accumulating too much moisture, one of the risk factors for recurrent vaginal yeast infections,' Peterson says."[77]

The wearing of thong underwear poses additional health concerns. According to Dr. Jill M. Rabin, "the string of a thong collects bacteria from your colon. The professor of OBGYN at Albert Einstein College of Medicine says that E.Coli is the most common type of bacteria in your colon. It accounts for 93% of UTIs but not a guarantee that you will contract a UTI when you wear a G-String. Wearing a satiny black thong puts you at a higher risk of UTI infections, Jill says.

"G-Strings carry the risk of causing external irritation. According to Dr. Shieva Ghofrany, an OBGYN with Stamford Hospital in Conn, most of her patients with skin tags near their vulva and rectum admit wearing thongs regularly. These skin tags result

---

[76] Susman, Carol, "Prevent Infections with Cotton Undies," Chicago Tribune. http://articles.chicagotribune.com/2006-12-27/features/0612270268_1_cotton-underwear-vaginal-undies

[77] Bowers, Elizabeth Shimer, "7 Surprising Benefits of Silk," Everyday Health. https://www.everydayhealth.com/skin-and-beauty-pictures/surprising-benefits-of-silk.aspx#05

from the skin being constantly rubbed in the same area. She notes that these happen traditionally at bra lines, but it is increasingly becoming popular at thong lines.

"According to Dr. Ghofanry, wearing thongs cannot cause hemorrhoid infections. But Dr. Harlan Wichelhaus, an OBGYN from the Specialty Obstetrics Gynecology and Fertility Department in Texas City, suggests otherwise. Dr. Wichelhaus indicates that wearing thongs regularly can trigger lacerations of the anus and in turn cause exacerbation of hemorrhoids."[78]

Perspiration is another factor to consider regarding our underwear. "Women and men who tend to sweat should change their underwear regularly — twice a day, as opposed to once a day for people who typically stay dry. And anyone who works out should put on a clean pair of undies as soon as they're able. 'A warm, moist environment is the perfect place for yeast to grow,' says Dr. [Donnica] Moore [a women's health expert], who recommends that sweat-prone people invest in underwear made of moisture-wicking material and avoid cotton underwear, which tends to stay wet once it gets wet. 'All of these problems are compounded if you have incontinence to any degree—even a drop or two,' says Dr. Moore. 'When you work out, you can try wearing a panty liner. That way, if you're not in a position to change underwear, at least you can change the panty liner or take it off.'"[79]

---

[78] Positive Med, "Ladies Only: 5 Reasons Not to Wear A Thong," Positive Med. http://positivemed.com/2016/12/25/not-wear-g-string/

[79] Schwartz, Sara, "8 Underwear Mistakes That Are Bad For Your Health," Huffington Post. https://www.huffingtonpost.com/entry/8-underwear-mistakes-that-are-bad-for-your-health_us_5602b6dbe4b00310edf95264

Now that we have highlighted the importance of carefully choosing our bras and underwear based on health factors, hopefully "out of sight" will not be "out of mind."

> *"Behold, You desire truth in the inward parts,*
> *And in the hidden part You will make me to know wisdom."*
> *Psalm 51:6, NKJV*

CHAPTER SIX

Footwear that "Kills" Your Feet

The Sixth Commandment

"You shall not kill."
Exodus 20: 13, NKJV

Principle

Avoid footwear that "kills" your feet and harms your body.

Proverbs 17:22 enlightens us to the fact that "a happy heart is good medicine and a cheerful mind works healing, but a broken spirit dries up the bones" (AMPC). Many centuries ago the wisest man that ever lived, King Solomon, wrote these words about the importance of a positive attitude, which today has been verified in many research studies. "The Mayo Clinic suggests that many health benefits have been influenced by a positive attitude, including increased life span, increased resistance to the common cold, lower rates of depression, increased cardiovascular health, reduced stress, and overall physical and mental vigor."[80]

Most women can attest to the challenge of maintaining a happy, cheerful attitude when many of the styles of footwear wreak

---

[80] Butler, Alia, "The Importance of Positive Attitude to Health," Livestrong. https://www.livestrong.com/article/126155-importance-positive-attitude-health/

havoc on our comfort and health. As we continue to consider our clothing's health effects, it can be helpful to understand the issues related to our fair footwear. With nearly 8,000 nerves in our feet, this can be a sensitive subject![81]

Many health articles, including those written by podiatrists, voice concerns about the effect of high heels upon the wearer. Podiatrist Leah Claydon is quoted in the book *Fashion Victim*: "For people who wear high heels more than a few times a week, the pain frequently goes beyond short-term problems like blisters and sore arches.... They'll typically notice that it becomes very hard to walk barefoot without getting pain in their calves."[82] The podiatrist states that the Achilles tendon shortens over time, "making it very difficult to put the heel to the floor when barefoot."[83]

Michelle Lee also illustrates the danger of high heels with several stories of tumbles, including an actress who "tumbled from four-inch high platforms and sprained her ankle and wrist while filming a TV show."[84]

Dr. William Rossi, a podiatrist, has published important details of the wearing of heels and their effect on our bodies. "Barefoot, the perpendicular line of the straight body column creates a ninety degree angle with the floor. On a two-inch heel, were the body a rigid column and forced to tilt forward, the angle would be reduced to seventy degrees, and to fifty-five degrees on a three-inch heel. Thus, for the body to maintain an erect position, a whole series of joint adjustments (ankle, knee, hip, spine, head) are required to regain and retain the erect stance.

---

[81] Foot, "Foot Facts," Foot. https://www.foot.com/foot-facts/
[82] Lee, Michelle (2003) *Fashion Victim*. New York: Broadway Books, 220.
[83] Ibid.
[84] Ibid, 221.

"But the alterations are internal and organic, as well. For example, when standing barefoot, the anterior angle of the female pelvis is twenty-five degrees; on low, one-inch heels it increases to thirty degrees; on two-inch heels to forty-five degrees; on three-inch heels to sixty degrees. Under these conditions, what happens to the pelvic and abdominal organs? Inevitably, these must shift position to adapt.

"Does the wearing of low, one-inch 'sensible' heels prevent these problems of postural adaptation? No. All the low heel does is lessen the intensity of the negative postural effects. Hence, the wearing of heels of any height automatically alters the natural erect state of the body column."[85]

One "study found walking in 3 1/2-inch heels causes more bone-on-bone movement in the knees than walking barefoot—researchers felt this may even explain why women have a higher incidence of osteoarthritis in the knees than men do."[86]

Not only high heels have adverse effects upon our precious health, but also flat shoes and even flip flop sandals. Both have been linked in research to plantar fasciitis. "The lack of arch support in ballet flats (or flat shoes of any sort, really) can wreak havoc on feet. To prevent plantar fasciitis, support and padding are equally necessary. Fortunately, arch supports can slip into most styles to make them more foot-friendly."[87]

---

[85] Rossi, William A., "Why Shoes Make 'Normal' Gait Impossible," Unshod. http://www.unshod.org/pfbc/pfrossi2.htm
[86] Fitzpatrick, Kelly, "14 Creepy Ways What You Wear Could Be Hurting Your Health," Greatist. http://greatist.com/health/14-health-risks-you-might-be-wearing
[87] Ibid.

In our personal search for well-fitting footwear, as well as absolutely every need in life, it is well worth the time to pray to our caring Heavenly Father and ask for His perfect guidance and provision. Poorly-fitting shoes can cause several problems. "Loose ones can cause corns and calluses, while too-tight shoes could cause bunions and in-grown toenails, not to mention painful swelling known as metatarsalgia."[88]

"Shoes that are too tight can cause long-term foot problems, says podiatrist Elizabeth Kurtz. Shop for shoes at the end of the day to compensate for foot swelling that occurs later in the day, and wear the same type of socks or hosiery you'll be wearing with the shoes. Choose a broad, rounded shoe with plenty of room for your toes and a wide, stable heel. Avoid pointy shoes, which can cramp your toes and cause ingrown toenails and calluses."[89]

Plastic surgeon Dr. Randal Haworth of Beverly Hills has developed Heel No Pain, a lidocaine spray. "With just a few quick sprays on foot aches, pains, burns, or itches, the topical liniment directly numbs the nerves that send pain signals to the brain. Heel No Pain/Style is considered to be a "painkiller with heat treatment" because it is able to penetrate while providing protective pain reflexes as the aches dissipate . . . Heel No Pain/Active is available for athletes who have real pain under their arch or experience tendinitis, sprains, and pulls. The unique analgesic spray has been developed for athletes to specifically target foot pain . . . With the combination of lidocaine HCl and tea tree oil to help treat and prevent athlete's foot, and peppermint oil to cool the burn, this

---

[88] Ibid.

[89] Sheehan, Jan, "10 Tips to Keep Your Feet Healthy," Everyday Health. https://www.everydayhealth.com/foot-health/tips-for-healthy-feet.aspx

version for athletes can help keep their endurance."[90] Dr. Anthony Weinert, a Michigan podiatrist, shares his concerns about the use of the spray. "Pain is an indicator that something is WRONG. As such, masking it means you're not getting the crucial signals of the damage being done, and you'll continue having damage done until the underlying cause is addressed."[91]

Foot odor and perspiration is an embarrassing problem for many. "There are [approximately] 250,000 sweat glands in a pair of feet. Sweat glands in the feet excrete as much as a half-pint of moisture a day."[92]

"Perspiration creates the perfect environment for bacteria to breed and ultimately leads to smelly feet. When dirt and sweat stay on your feet too long, they can even lead to athlete's foot and other foot infections . . . change your socks daily to prevent foot odor [and] allow your feet to breathe by taking your shoes off after you get home."[93]

There are differing recommendations regarding the best fibers for socks for health. Some believe that one should "always wear cotton socks and avoid wearing socks made of synthetic fibers

---

[90] Borreli, Lizette, "'Heel No Pain,' Foot-Numbing Spray, Eliminates High Heel Aches," Medical Daily. http://www.medicaldaily.com/heel-no-pain-foot-numbing-spray-eliminates-high-heel-aches-lidocaine-hci-deadens-foot-pain-3-hours

[91] Weinert, Anthony, "'Heel No Pain' Lidocaine Sprain: Numbing Your Pain Doesn't Fix Your Pain," Dr. Anthony Weinert. http://dranthonyweinert.com/heel-no-pain-lidocaine-sprain/

[92] Foot, "Foot Facts," Foot. https://www.foot.com/foot-facts/

[93] Top 10 Home Remedies, "10 Foot Care Tips that You Must Follow," Top 10 Home Remedies. http://www.top10homeremedies.com/news-facts/10-foot-care-tips-that-you-must-follow.html

as well as excessively tight pantyhose, which trap moisture."[94] Others state that "the best fabrics for antifungal socks are merino wool, Coolmax, olefin, Drymax and polyester. If you play a ton of sports, or even just wear shoes for long periods of time where your feet get sweaty, consider these socks to avoid fungal infections. Always remember, dry feet are healthy feet!"[95]

Not only affecting those athletically inclined, it is important to note that "Athlete's foot, also called tinea pedis, is a fungal infection of the foot. It causes peeling, redness, itching, burning, and sometimes blisters and sores.

"Athlete's foot is a very common infection. The fungus grows best in a warm, moist environment such as shoes, socks, swimming pools, locker rooms, and the floors of public showers. It is most common in the summer and in warm, humid climates. It occurs more often in people who wear tight shoes and who use community baths and pools.[96]

According to Elizabeth Kurtz, DPM, a podiatrist in Chicago and spokesperson for the American Podiatric Medical Association (APMA), the following recommendations will help keep your prized peds healthier:

- **Protect your feet in public areas.** Be sure to wear shower shoes at the gym, in locker rooms, and at public pools. These places tend to be breeding grounds for fungi that can lead to infections.

---

[94] Ibid.

[95] The Soxperts, "Best Anti-fungal Socks," Socks Addict. https://www.socksaddict.com/blog/best-anti-fungal-socks/

[96] WebMD, "Fungal Infections of the Skin," WebMD. https://www.webmd.com/skin-problems-and-treatments/guide/fungal-infections-skin#1

- **Avoid sharing footgear.** "You can get fungal infections by wearing other people's shoes, as well as socks worn by another person," says Kurtz. This includes rentals. Always wear your own footgear to help keep your feet healthy.
- **Head off sweaty feet.** Your feet have sweat glands galore — 250,000 in each foot! Perspiration creates the perfect environment for bacteria to set up shop. Wearing socks that keep feet dry will help your feet stay healthy. "Socks made of synthetic fibers tend to wick away moisture faster than cotton or wool socks," says Kurtz. Also avoid wearing excessively tight pantyhose, which trap moisture.
- **Choose breathable footwear.** To help keep your feet dry and healthy, wear shoes made of leather to allow air to circulate. If you're prone to excessively sweaty feet, look for shoes made of mesh fabrics for maximum breathability.[97]

As we choose footwear for our healthy clothes closet, let us remember the joy of comfortable feet as well as the potential health benefits of proper footwear.

"How beautiful are thy feet with shoes, O prince's daughter!"
Song of Solomon 7:1

---

[97] Sheehan, Jan, "10 Tips to Keep Your Feet Healthy," Everyday Health. https://www.everydayhealth.com/foot-health/tips-for-healthy-feet.aspx

CHAPTER SEVEN

Posture and Purses

The Seventh Commandment

"You shall not commit adultery."
Exodus 20:14, NKJV

Principle

Do not adulterate your posture with unhealthy purses.

The Scriptures encourage us to "each one . . . bear [her] own load" (Galatians 6:5, NKJV). While the faultless biblical principle is true that we should carry our own responsibilities, we women may carry, on a regular basis, excess weight in our pretty purses that contributes to pain and suffering. Add to this the weight of a laptop attaché or diaper bag, and it becomes imperative that we carefully evaluate the beloved handbags we carry.

"According to the American Chiropractic Association, half of working Americans admit to having back pain. What's more, our nation as a whole is spending at least *$50 billion* each year to remedy that pain. One culprit? Our heavy purses."[98]

---

[98] Adams, Rebecca, "Why Your Purse Is Giving You Back Pain," Huffington Post.

"It's easy to dismiss the 'pocketbook effect' but when you carry something heavy every day, the accumulated stress can lead to significant injuries that require medical attention," says Martin Lanoff, MD, a physical medicine and rehabilitation specialist and a clinical assistant professor at Rosalind Franklin University Medical School in Chicago.[99]

"One of the consequences of carrying a shoulder bag on one shoulder is that it significantly interferes with the normal gait," says Dr. Karen Erickson, a New York-based chiropractor.[100] The swinging of our arms and legs when we walk naturally is an important way to keep our body balanced. When we have a handbag on one side of the body, the arm on that side cannot swing properly and the other arm will compensate with an exaggerated swing.

When all of the weight of our bag is on one shoulder, we're carrying an asymmetric load, which throws off our posture. Most of us tend to carry purses on our side of dominance. But this causes the muscles in our dominant shoulder, particularly the trapezius muscle, to become larger. "We see asymmetry in posture—like, one shoulder's higher than the other—from this chronic forcing of the

---

https://www.huffingtonpost.com/2013/12/09/purse-back-pain_n_4397727.html

[99] Shaffer, Alyssa, "Is Your Purse Wrecking Your Back?," Prevention. https://www.prevention.com/health/health-concerns/bags-and-back-pain-could-your-purse-or-handbag-be-causing-pain

[100] Adams, Rebecca, "Why Your Purse Is Giving You Back Pain," Huffington Post. https://www.huffingtonpost.com/2013/12/09/purse-back-pain_n_4397727.html

muscles on one side to become more developed than the muscles on the other side," Dr. Erickson states.[101]

"This asymmetric load also causes muscles in your spine to compensate for the weight, which can cause the opposite side of the spine to go into spasm'" adds Dr. Robert Hayden, a chiropractor and founder of The Iris City Chiropractic Center in Atlanta. This overcompensation can also affect the lower back and sacrum. The more asymmetric the load, the more everything below the shoulder will have to work.[102]

These concerns are verified in a study published in the *Journal of Physical Therapy Science*. Using a gait analyzer, right-handed female subjects were "instructed to walk while carrying a bag, which weighted approximately 10% of the subjects' average weight, in four different ways; holding it in the left hand, carrying it over the left shoulder, holding it in the right hand, and carrying it over the right shoulder. Subjects who habitually carried bags on their right exhibited changes in gait variables related to walking distance. In addition, their gait velocities were relatively faster. On the other hand, differences in temporal and spatial gait variables were not exhibited when the bag was carried using the four methods."[103] The researchers concluded that when the weight of a bag is appropriate, bag-carrying habits did have significant effects on gait. It is important for those who carry bags to avoid the habit of carrying them on only one side.[104]

---

[101] Ibid.

[102] Ibid.

[103] Son, SungMin and Hyolyun Noh, "Gait Changes Caused By the Habits and Methods of Carrying a Handbag," *Journal of Physical Therapy Science*, NCBI, NLM.
https://www.ncbi.nlm.nih.gov/pmc/articles/PMC3820208/

[104] Ibid.

Carrying a heavy purse adds additional concerns. It can cause the trapezius muscle at the top of our shoulders to spasm and therefore tighten, along with the muscles that go from the shoulder to the base of the neck. "When that happens, it can cause a lot of stiffness in the upper back, the shoulder area and the neck," says Dr. Erickson. It can also cause a decreased curve in the neck, which is known as "military neck."

"We also see people who develop arthritis in their neck, in their lower neck, because their neck has been forced to carry this heavy weight for such a long period of time," says Dr. Erickson. The delicate muscles that help us carry our purses also assist with turning our heads, making that action painful.

Some individuals will develop tension headaches from the muscles being forced to do all of this heavy lifting, says Dr. Erickson. When the muscles in our shoulder and neck area spasm, it can cause pain in the back of our skulls that radiates around to the front.[105]

Additional health issues which may be caused or exacerbated by carrying a too-heavy bag are scoliosis ("S" curvature of the spine) or kyphosis (hunchback) in women with weak bones, and numbness and tingling in the arm from nerve microtrauma.[106]

In determining how much weight is too much, these guidelines are offered by Toronto physiotherapist Angela Growse. "The weight of a backpack when loaded should be no more than 15 percent of your body weight. So, for a woman who is 140 pounds, that's 21 pounds maximum. A handbag should be five to eight percent of body weight (so seven to 11 pounds for a 140-pound

---

[105] Ibid.

[106] Shaffer, Alyssa, "Is Your Purse Wrecking Your Back?," Prevention. https://www.prevention.com/health/health-concerns/bags-and-back-pain-could-your-purse-or-handbag-be-causing-pain

individual). And it doesn't take much to go over the ideal weight, considering a leather laptop case weighs up to seven pounds without a laptop in it."[107]

According to the American Chiropractic Association, a bag should weigh no more than 10 percent of your body weight. Dr. Karen Erikson, who is a spokeswoman for the American Chiropractic Association, recommends not exceeding 5 percent with purses.[108]

With the need to keep our purse weight as low as possible, we must carefully consider the style of bag we carry. Some bags have heavy hardware, such as metal chains, buckles and large zipper pulls. Leather is heavier than fabric or nylon. "If you choose leather, the more important thing is to keep the load close to your body," states Ms. Growse.[109]

She provides several guidelines for choosing a healthy handbag. "A backpack with padded straps and a waist belt is optimal, 'because the weight is distributed primarily onto the hips,' says Ms. Growse, who acknowledges that a backpack isn't for everyone, every day. 'Obviously, for work you want to choose something that is appropriate,' she says. Next best for the body? A

---

[107] Best Health Magazine, "How to Choose a Healthy Handbag," Reader's Digest Best Health. http://www.besthealthmag.ca/best-looks/beauty/how-to-choose-a-healthy-handbag/

[108] Clayton, Jaimie Dalessio, "5 Unhealthy Handbag Habits," Everyday Health. https://www.everydayhealth.com/pain-management-pictures/unhealthy-handbag-habits.aspx#01

[109] Best Health Magazine, "How to Choose a Healthy Handbag," Reader's Digest Best Health. http://www.besthealthmag.ca/best-looks/beauty/how-to-choose-a-healthy-handbag/

padded-strap cross-body bag (any bag with a long or adjustable strap that allows you to wear it across the body). The cross-body rates high because it's 'stable and secure, and leaves the hands and arms free.' Third best is a shoulder bag with a wide padded strap (or with two 'rolled' straps). 'Carrying a bag in the crook of your arm might be a popular look, but it's 'mechanically poor,' Ms. Growse says. 'You're scrunching your shoulder, causing compression between neck and shoulder.'"[110]

Dr. Erickson suggests using a handbag with small, briefcase-style handles that you hold in your hand instead of sliding onto your shoulder. Messenger bags and other cross body styles are also good at distributing weight. "Thin-strapped bags, especially ones that are too heavy, can cut into the shoulder muscle, causing pain. Metal straps can worsen that pain. Thicker straps better distribute the weight." She also cautions that if you decide to wear a backpack in order to evenly distribute the weight, be sure you're wearing it properly. To start, use both backpack straps instead of sliding it onto one shoulder. Also make sure the backpack doesn't hang too low down your back. Ideally it should be at the bottom of the rib cage, Dr. Erickson says, not by your waist.[111]

"Hold your bag on your shoulder—not in the crook of your arm. This way you'll avoid elbow injuries like tendinitis," Dr. Lanoff states. Also, limit strain by carrying two small bags instead of one heavy one.[112]

---

[110] Ibid.

[111] Adams, Rebecca, "Why Your Purse Is Giving You Back Pain," Huffington Post. https://www.huffingtonpost.com/2013/12/09/purse-back-pain_n_4397727.html

[112] Shaffer, Alyssa, "Is Your Purse Wrecking Your Back?," Prevention. https://www.prevention.com/health/health-

"You'll want to switch sides every block or two that you walk," says Dr. Erickson. "Most of us have a side and we do it for 20 years, 30 years and the reason is that it's comfortable," she says. But it helps to get in the habit of switching sides. "I recommend if someone is out and about for the day with a bag, and your shoulder ends up hurting, pull it in front of you like a baby so you get it off your shoulders for a while," says Dr. Erickson. Stretching, light weights and other forms of exercise can help ensure that your shoulders are equally strong and toned. It's also helpful to simply try walking without a bag from time to time to restore that natural gait, Dr. Erickson says. "When you go out for lunch, for example, just carry essentials, like credit cards, and walk with your arms swinging," she says. "You don't even need to exaggerate the swing; just a natural swing is really very good for the shoulders."[113]

Dr. Erikson has two other important recommendations. "Avoid hauling the same big bag everywhere you go. Getting the habit of doing so, and you'll only keep adding to its bulk as the days pass. Keep a separate bag for the gym, or for extra shoes, instead of loading it all up inside one massive tote." In addition, "Make sure the bag fits. Believe it or not, some bags might not fit you the right way. "Get the height of the bag to match your sweet spot," says Erickson. "If it's too short you can't swing your arms, and if it's too long it messes up your gait. The bag should hit right around your waist."[114]

Heidi Prather, an associate professor of physical medicine and rehabilitation at the Washington University School of Medicine, in St. Louis, advises us to "make a conscious effort to keep both

---

concerns/bags-and-back-pain-could-your-purse-or-handbag-be-causing-pain
[113] Ibid.
[114] Ibid.

shoulders pulled down and level. 'Many women instinctively lift and tense the shoulder that has the handbag on it,' says Ms. Prather. This only exacerbates the tendency to have short, weak muscles between the shoulder blades, which can be the first to flare up. If you talk on your cell phone while carrying a bulky bag, your neck and back will be doubly stressed by the ear-to-shoulder muscle tension. A wireless headset for walking and talking is a better option.[115]

In an article in *Prevention,* it was recommended to "put your purse on a diet." Four common areas of weight accumulation are wallets, key chains, coupons and makeup. Routinely evaluating and removing unnecessary items can greatly reduce purse weight. Take out change, remove keys not used daily, cull expired or unused coupons and pare down cosmetics carried.[116]

Julie Morgenstern, author of *Organizing From the Inside Out,* has several suggestions for reducing the weight and bulk of our bags. "She recommends to spend a few minutes in the evening sorting out the next day's schedule. Noontime workout? Big event after work? 'Know exactly what's on your plate so you don't weigh yourself down carrying unnecessary items,' Ms. Morgenstern says." She also suggests to divide our purse into two sections, one area with permanent items used daily, and the second area with temporary items, cleaned out nightly to avoid carrying what we do not need. Ms. Morgenstern also encourages a pouch system, using zippered bags that can be added or removed on an as-needed basis. Examples

---

[115] Sullivan, Dana, "How to Lighten a Heavy Purse," Real Simple. https://www.realsimple.com/health/preventative-health/aches-pains/heavy-purse#declutter-you-purse-daily

[116] Shaffer, Alyssa, "Is Your Purse Wrecking Your Back?," Prevention. https://www.prevention.com/health/health-concerns/bags-and-back-pain-could-your-purse-or-handbag-be-causing-pain

include bags for makeup, change, coupons and pens and a small notebook. Another idea is to have a small spare handbag that fits just the essentials (wallet, cell phone, keys) to take when traveling a short distance.[117]

Lead toxicity risk is an additional concern for our pretty purses. A report from the nonprofit Center for Environmental Health (CEH) found that many inexpensive faux-leather bags sold at department stores and discount retailers have toxic levels of lead, some up to 90 times higher than the federal limit for lead in paint. The purses were made of PVC, vinyl or polyurethane. Yellow bags had the highest lead levels, although all colors tested were positive for lead. Recommendations include purchasing bags of other materials and keeping children away from bags made from these synthetic materials.[118]

We lovely ladies might be appalled if we knew the germs our purses can carry. "Bags travel just as much as we do—from the bedroom to the car (or the train), then the office or the grocery store, then a restaurant or bar, even a public bathroom, then back home to the kitchen counter. You get the idea. Beyond making your bag look dirty faster, placing it on the floor can collect bacteria, like staph and E. coli, which can cause infection. Avoid putting your bag in these places and wipe it down daily.[119]

---

[117] Ibid.

[118] Main, Emily, "Your Purse May Be Contaminated with Toxic Metal," Rodale Wellness. https://www.rodalewellness.com/health/lead-and-purses

[119] Clayton, Jaimie Dalessio, "5 Unhealthy Handbag Habits," Everyday Health. https://www.everydayhealth.com/pain-management-pictures/unhealthy-handbag-habits.aspx#01

We women have a two-fold consideration for our purses: health-aiding style as well as wise weight management of the contents. "People really want to create a certain look, and handbags are a way to say a lot about you in a glance" Dr. Erickson says. "But I think it's important to prioritize your health above all else."[120] Thankfully our kind Heavenly Father, Who "make[s] known the end from the beginning" (Isaiah 46:10, NIV), can guide us to find the perfect purse for our lifestyle as well as what we do and do not need to carry for each day's demands.

> *"If any of you lacks wisdom [to guide (her) through a decision or circumstance], [she] is to ask of [our benevolent] God, who gives to everyone generously and without rebuke or blame, and it will be given to [her]."*
> James 1:5, AMP

---

[120] Adams, Rebecca, "Why Your Purse Is Giving You Back Pain," Huffington Post. https://www.huffingtonpost.com/2013/12/09/purse-back-pain_n_4397727.html

CHAPTER EIGHT

Fabrics and Health

The Eighth Commandment

"You shall not steal."
Exodus 20: 15, NKJV

Principle

Do not let the fabrics you wear steal your health.

Beautiful, feminine fabrics are a delight to our eyes, and they also can be a blessing to our health. In the Holy Bible, there are three fabrics stated as used for clothing: linen (Exodus 28:39), silk (Ezekiel 16:10), and wool, specifically lambswool (Proverbs 27:26). These natural fabrics, as well as cotton, are health-promoting clothing options for those without sensitivities.

It is interesting that our wise Lord has instructed us to "not wear a garment of different sorts, such as wool and linen mixed together" (Deuteronomy 22:11). This is due to the difference in the effects of the fabrics upon the skin—they act as opposites. Our wonderful Creator does not want our skin in confusion any more than He would want our minds confused. Whereas wool is insulating for warmth and moisture-wicking,[121] linen is cooling because it absorbs heat and moisture and evaporates it quickly.[122]

Wool

A classic fiber obtained from shearing sheep, wool has many health benefits. Wool is a breathable fabric often preferred in winter because it is a "great buffer against rain, wind and snow. The scientific reasons for these 'miraculous' properties are that, in cold temperatures, wool removes (wicks) moisture from the skin whilst at the same time its insulating qualities trap dry air and warmth."[123] Wool is naturally water-resistant, so that our bodies can stay warm even when the fabric is damp. "So if you're wearing wooly socks and get water in your wellies [rubber boots], your feet will feel much less cold or damp. Added to that, wool's unique structure means that it won't allow the build-up of body odours."[124] These are several reasons that outer garments as well as high performance base layers are made of wool. Soft yet strong, merino wool is preferred by some next to their skin.

Many practical-minded women and men appreciate wool. Wool is "easy to clean because dirt sits on the surface of the fibre (and so can be wiped off), it needs very little washing or laundry. It dries

---

[121] Greco, Jeremiah, "Wool vs. Cotton: When and Where" Orvis News http://www.orvis.com/news/products-we-love/wool-vs-cotton-when-and-where/

[122] LinenMe, "Benefits of Wearing Linen Clothes in Summer," LinenMe https://www.linenme.com/news/benefits-of-wearing-linen-clothes-in-summer/

[123] The Wool Company, "The Benefits of Wool," The Wool Company, England. https://www.thewoolcompany.co.uk/benefits-of-wool.html

[124] Ibid.

quickly and is flame-retardant. Naturally anti-allergenic, wool doesn't collect static which attracts dust and dirt."[125]

What about the individuals who state they have a wool allergy? It turns out that the scratchy sensation some experience when wearing wool is not a true allergic reaction, because the immune system is not activated. "People report any fabric as being scratchy and irritating when it has over 5% of its fibers thicker than 30 microns in diameter. Many sheep's wools have fibers in this range. But scientists have duplicated the sensation with artificial fibers such as nylon, proving that the skin irritation is not specific to wool. . . . Fine Merino wool is about 18 microns and therefore unlikely to produce a scratchy feeling. Cashmere, from Cashmere goats, ranges from about 14 microns to about 18."[126]

For those who truly have an allergic reaction to wool, there are several potential causes and solutions. "If you are concerned about wool allergies, it is believed that people who suffer from wool allergies are allergic to chemicals in wool, not the wool itself. Using organic or eco wool may alleviate the problem."[127] Others may find that their allergy to wool is actually caused by lanolin, the oily sebum found in a sheep's fleece. "Symptoms of exposure are a red skin rash, which may be accompanied by a runny nose, sneezing, breathing problems and conjunctivitis (red eyes) . . . If you are allergic to lanolin, you may experience the same reaction when exposed to

---

[125] Ibid.

[126] Pelletier, T.C., "Lanolin and Sheep's Wool Allergies," Ask a Naturalist. http://askanaturalist.com/lanolin-and-sheep%E2%80%99s-wool-allergies/

[127] Webb, Irina, "A Quick Guide to Amazing Wool Health Benefits," I Read Labels For You. https://ireadlabelsforyou.com/amazing-wool-health-benefits/

cosmetic creams, waxes and other products containing it; sufferers have reported problems with sheep-derived vitamin D and air fresheners containing lanolin compounds."[128] The good news for those who love the benefits of wool but cannot wear it is that "most other animals, such as alpacas, llamas, cashmere goats and angora rabbits, do not have lanolin in their wool, so wearing those fibres is fine!"[129]

Research studies also confirm the health benefits of wearing wool. "Consistent with earlier science findings, the early results from a study undertaken by the University of Sydney, Australia, are showing that wool sleeping apparel and bedding increases total sleep time, promotes sleep onset and improves sleep efficiency.

"In hot (29° Celsius) conditions, wearing wool sleepwear saw participants in the study sleep significantly longer, reflecting faster sleep onset and waking up less frequently. In both cold (17° Celsius) and neutral (22° Celsius) conditions, the combination of wool sleepwear and bedding saw participants have a more efficient sleep compared to when tested using non-wool sleepwear and bedding."[130]

Another study found pain relief for fibromyalgia patients through the use of wool. "The patients in the treatment group wore woolen underwear (which covered the body from the shoulders to the thighs) and used woolen bedding such as woolen bed liner, woolen quilt and pillow during the experimental period of 6 weeks. . . . Patients in the treatment group reported significant improvements in their conditions including a reduction in pain

---

[128] Serena, "Wool Allergies: Their Causes and Effects," Love Knitting. https://blog.loveknitting.com/wool-allergies/
[129] Ibid.
[130] Woolmark, "Benefits of Wool," Woolmark. https://www.woolmark.com/resources/benefits-of-wool/

levels, tender point counts, and all scores of the Fibromyalgia Impact Questionnaire.

"The use of woolen underwear and woolen bedding were effective in reducing the symptoms of patients suffering from fibromyalgia. The use of wool is recommended as a means of treatment for alleviating the pain of fibromyalgia."[131]

Cotton

Cotton, a plant fiber made into fabric, is not only health-promoting but it also is very practical and economical. "The world uses cotton more than any other natural fiber and it is primarily grown and used to make cloth."[132] "Cotton clothing protects against from heat in the summer and cold in the winter by providing thermal insulation as the cotton fabric traps air between the fabric fibers. The cotton fibers in clothing hold the fabric away from the skin, further allowing for more air to be trapped between the skin and fabric which helps with insulation and comfort."[133] Cotton also lets heat escape, but holds moisture next to the skin once damp.[134]

---

[131] Kiyak, E.K., "A New Nonpharmacological Method in Fibromyalgia: The Use of Wool," Journal of Alternative Complementary Medicine, NCBI, NLM.
https://www.ncbi.nlm.nih.gov/pubmed/19388862

[132] Peterman, William, "The Advantages of Cotton Clothing," Livestrong.
https://www.livestrong.com/article/59826-advantages-cotton-clothing/

[133] Ibid.

[134] Greco, Jeremiah, "Wool vs. Cotton: When and Where," Orvis.
http://www.orvis.com/news/products-we-love/wool-vs-cotton-when-and-where/

"Cotton is soft, absorbent and breathable. So, if your clothes are itchy, irritating, stiff or clingy,"[135] consider cotton instead. Regarding static cling, "cotton is never the culprit because it can't hold an electric charge."[136]

Cotton fabric rarely causes allergic reactions; in fact, wearing cotton is often recommended for those with skin allergies, notes Cotton Incorporated. "Because cotton is hypoallergenic [it] does not irritate skin."[137] For those who do have reactions to cotton clothing, there is the option (albeit expensive) of organic clothing. Organic cotton has the ability to be worn by people with chemical sensitivities because it does not contain the dyes and traces of chemicals found in conventional cotton.[138]

Silk

Silk thread is obtained from the cocoons of moth larvae. Each larva spins about a kilometer [about two-thirds of a mile] of thread![139] This beautiful fabric also has health benefits. "Silk is a natural heat regulator, maintaining the correct body temperature. It does not conduct heat or static electricity like other fibers. Heat is retained during cold temperatures and redundant heat is shed during warm

---

[135] The Fabric of Our Lives, "The Benefits of Cotton," Cotton Inc. https://thefabricofourlives.com/learn-about-cotton/the-benefits-of-cotton

[136] Ibid.

[137] Ibid.

[138] Organic Lifestyle, "Organic Cotton—Why Bother?," Organic Lifestyle. https://organiclifestyle.com/organic-cotton/organic-cotton-why-bother?currency_code=USD

[139] Melissa, "How Is Silk Made?," Today I Found Out. http://www.todayifoundout.com/index.php/2014/10/real-silk-made/

temperatures, keeping your skin cool in the summer and warm in the winter."[140]

"Multiple studies have pointed to the antimicrobial properties of a special European silk fabric called DermaSilk," states Jennifer Peterson, MD, a dermatologist at the Dermatology & Laser Surgery Center in Houston.[141] Dermasilk differs from regular silk in that it's free of sericin, a protein produced by the silkworm which may aggravate eczema and other skin conditions. "One particular study showed improvements in patients with the skin condition eczema who used Dermasilk, but not in those who used cotton," she adds.[142]

"People are very rarely allergic to silk," says Neal B. Schultz, MD, a New York City dermatologist. This is because silk is free of any potentially irritating added chemicals and contains natural substances that ward off various environmental allergens (and resulting skin conditions), including dust mites, mold, and fungus, he explains."[143]

Linen

Linen is a strong fiber woven from the flax plant. It is commonly worn in hot weather for its benefit of facilitating the

---

[140] Sleep N' Beauty, "The Real Benefits of Sleeping on Silk," Sleep N' Beauty.
https://sleepnbeauty.com/blogs/news/13894827-the-real-benefits-of-sleeping-on-silk

[141] Bowers, Elizabeth Shimer, "7 Surprising Benefits of Silk," Everyday Health.
https://www.everydayhealth.com/skin-and-beauty-pictures/surprising-benefits-of-silk.aspx#06

[142] Ibid.

[143] Ibid.

cooling of the body. Clothes made of linen possess high air permeability, which allows air to flow through the fabric easily and allows the body to breathe.[144]

Another benefit of linen clothing is keeping the body free of moisture due to its high absorbency. Linen garments feels cool to the touch, absorbing moisture and removing perspiration from the skin, and then quickly releasing it again. This is a great asset for our bodies' detoxification through our sweat glands. "Because of its molecular structure linen cloth can absorb as much as 1/5 of its weight before giving a feeling of being damp or wet."[145]

Linen also has excellent heat conductivity characteristics. "Heat conductivity refers to the extent to which heat can be conveyed through the fabric. As linen quickly allows the heat to escape, it further improves cooling. It is claimed that heat conductivity of linen is five times higher than wool and eighteen times higher than silk."[146]

Linen can be helpful for some with specific health concerns. Linen fabric is naturally resistant to fungus and bacteria; this has been found to be a benefit for some who have skin rashes and eczema. Allergic reactions are not found from wearing linen, and can be helpful in treating a number of allergic disorders. In addition, since linen provides a healthy air exchange and heat conductivity, it can be useful in reducing fever.[147]

---

[144] LinenMe, "Benefits of Wearing Linen Clothes in Summer," LinenMe.
https://www.linenme.com/news/benefits-of-wearing-linen-clothes-in-summer/
[145] Ibid.
[146] Ibid.
[147] Ibid.

Linen has not been found to accumulate static electricity. "Even a small addition of flax fibers (up to 10%) to a cloth is enough to eliminate the static electricity effect. It possesses high air permeability and heat. Heat conductivity of linen is five times as high as wool and 19 times that of silk. In hot weather those dressed in linen clothing are found to show skin temperatures 3-4 degrees C below that of their silk or cotton-wearing friends. According to some studies, a person wearing linen clothes perspires 1.5 times less than when dressed in cotton clothes, and twice less than when dressed in viscose [rayon] clothes."[148]

It is very interesting that Dr. Philip Callahan, a physician and researcher, "found that when the pure flax cloth was put over a wound or local pain, it greatly accelerated the healing process."[149] One woman reported she wore linen underwear to help with yeast infections and found that her chronic hip pain was relieved.[150]

Synthetics

There are many consumers who are concerned about using synthetic fabrics, such as nylon, for clothing. Many synthetic fabrics do not "breathe" and allow perspiration to evaporate, making them uncomfortable and unhealthy. Another concern with synthetic fabrics is the toxicity of the chemicals used. According to the Underground Health Reporter, "Health complications associated with skin contact with the toxic chemicals in synthetic clothing

---

[148] Norton, Rosemary, "Properties of Linen," Linen 4 Life. http://www.linen4life.net/properties--care.html

[149] Life-giving Linen, "Scientific Details of the Linen Frequency Study," Life-giving Linen. http://www.lifegivinglinen.com/linen-study.html

[150] Life-giving Linen, "Underwear Testimonials," Life-giving Linen. http://www.lifegivinglinen.com/organic-linen-underwear.html

include infertility, respiratory diseases, contact dermatitis and cancer, to name just a few."[151] Formaldehyde, linked to an increase in lung cancer in research, can be found in fabrics that are labeled as anti-cling, anti-static, anti-shrink, waterproof, or moth-proof and mildew resistant.[152]

Unfortunately, natural fabrics are not free from toxicity issues. "Keep in mind that many fabrics (including natural fibers) undergo significant processing that often involves detergents, petrochemical dyes, formaldehyde to prevent shrinkage, volatile organic compounds (VOCs), dioxin-producing bleach and chemical fabric softeners. These additives are often toxic to the human body, may contain heavy metals and can pollute our environment."[153] Organic clothing is offered as the best option when seeking to avoid adding to one's toxic overload. "While they still might be processed to some extent, they are often a better choice than synthetics."[154]

While some conscientious individuals wear only natural fabrics and no synthetics, others use both as they deem appropriate. Dr. Agatha Thrash suggested that "nylon and many other synthetics are satisfactory for top clothing or overclothing, and may, if the knit is bulky, be suitable for protective sports dress and underclothing. In

---

[151] Underground Health Reporter, "Fact or Myth: Are Clothes Made with Synthetic Fibers Toxic Clothing and Hazardous to Your Health?" Underground Health Reporter.
http://undergroundhealthreporter.com/toxic-clothing-synthetic-fibers-hazard-to-health/
[152] Ibid.
[153] Body Ecology, "6 Fabrics You Should Avoid Wearing and Why," Body Ecology.
https://bodyecology.com/articles/top_6_fabrics_you_should_avoid_wearing.php
[154] Ibid.

warm weather, [most] synthetics cling to moisture and trap body heat, making them unsatisfactory for summer wear."[155]

Many physically active women are finding that the newer synthetic active wear can be advantageous even in warm weather. "This is because the new generation of technical fabrics are created to allow moisture through the weave and wick away from the body, where it can evaporate on the surface, keeping you cool. Technical fabrics can also be waterproof. It may sound like a contradiction, but some fabrics can be both breathable and waterproof, allowing you to get caught in a downpour but not feel steamy inside after a few hours of hiking."[156]

Dr. Thrash stated that "absorptive cotton for underclothing, not synthetic fabrics, are often required to meet all the various needs of the body."[157] Her concern regarding synthetic underwear finds others in agreement. Jaimie Clayton reports that "synthetic materials like nylon and Lycra can also cause problems when used in underwear. Unlike breathable cotton, these fabrics keep in moisture and heat — providing a breeding ground for yeast infections."[158]

---

[155] Thrash, Agatha, "Healthful Body Temperature," Uchee Pines. http://www.ucheepines.org/healthful-body-temperature/

[156] Fehr, Melissa, "A Guide to Activewear Fabrics," Seamwork. https://www.seamwork.com/issues/2015/01/a-guide-to-activewear-fabrics

[157] Thrash, Agatha, "Clothing," Uchee Pines. http://www.ucheepines.org/clothing/

[158] Clayton, Jaimie Dalessio, "5 Ways Clothing Can Make You Sick," Everyday Health. http://www.everydayhealth.com/pain-management-pictures/ways-clothing-can-make-you-sick.aspx#06

Another concern about synthetic clothing is static cling. Static electricity, its health effects and methods to reduce it will be discussed in Chapter Nine.

Whether we choose clothing sewn from natural or synthetic fabrics, our faithful Heavenly Father promises to guide us to make the best choice for our health and to provide all our wardrobe needs. "If God dresses grass in the field so beautifully, even though it's alive today and tomorrow it's thrown into the furnace, won't God do much more for you, you people of weak faith?" (Matthew 6:30, CEB).

"But first and most importantly seek (aim at, strive after)
His kingdom and His righteousness
[His way of doing and being right—the attitude and character of God],
and all these things [food, clothing] will be given to you also."
Matthew 6:33, AMP

CHAPTER NINE

Cleanliness and Health

The Ninth Commandment

"You shall not bear false witness against your neighbor."
Exodus 20: 16, NKJV

Principle

Do not bear a false witness of cleanliness by allowing toxins to remain on clothing.

The phrase "cleanliness is next to godliness" is not found in the sacred Scriptures. Nonetheless, it is true that comely cleanliness is extremely important, not only for our environment and personal hygiene, but also for our attractive clothing.

"God commanded that the children of Israel should in no case allow impurities of their persons, or of their clothing. Those who had any personal uncleanness were shut out of the camp until evening, and then were required to cleanse themselves and their clothing before they could enter the camp [Leviticus 11, 15].

"In regard to cleanliness, God requires no less of his people now, than he did of ancient Israel. A neglect of cleanliness will induce disease. Sickness and premature death, do not come without a cause."[159]

"Impurities are constantly and imperceptibly passing from the body, through the pores, and if the surface of the skin is not kept in a healthy condition, the system is burdened with impure matter. If the clothing worn is not often washed, and frequently aired, it becomes filthy with impurities which are thrown off from the body by sensible and insensible perspiration. And if the garments worn are not frequently cleansed from these impurities, the pores of the skin absorb again the waste matter thrown off. The impurities of the body, if not allowed to escape, are taken back into the blood, and forced upon the internal organs. Nature, to relieve herself of poisonous impurities, makes an effort to free the system, which effort produces fevers."[160]

Regarding laundering of clothing, it is best to always wash the clothing we have purchased before wearing. This is necessary whether the clothing purchased is new or used. New clothing can contain toxic chemicals such as synthetic dyes or formaldehyde resin, which can lead to contact dermatitis or other conditions. According to an interview with a dermatologist published in *The Wall Street Journal*, washing new items and rinsing twice is recommended before wearing.[161]

If clothing is used, there can be micro-organisms, toxins, or cosmetics from the previous owner which need cleansed. According

---

[159] White, E. G. (1958). *Selected Messages Book 2*. Washington, D.C.: Review and Herald Publishing Association. 461.

[160] White, E. G. (1958). *Selected Messages Book 2*. Washington, D.C.: Review and Herald Publishing Association. 460.

[161] Mitchell, Heidi, "Do You Need to Wash New Clothes Before Wearing Them?" The Wall Street Journal.

to author Michelle Lee, most thrift stores in the U.S. do not launder donated apparel because it is cost prohibitive.[162]

Some laundry detergents can cause contact dermatitis, so it behooves us to carefully observe our lovely skin. According to Dr. Donnica Moore, a women's health expert, "The No. 1 cause of [unexplained itching in our private areas] is your laundry detergent. The tissues that your panties come in to contact with are a lot more sensitive than your elbows."[163] Sensitive individuals may find that they are able to tolerate perfume and dye-free commercial laundry detergents. There are also many recipes on the internet for inexpensive, homemade laundry soap, which can be less irritating for some. In addition, "clothing dye is a common cause of allergic skin rash," says allergist Neeta Ogden, M.D., "especially blue and orange dyes in clothing and other items." Elastics on socks, underwear and bras can also cause rashes in some people because of the rubber, she says. Particularly if you find you react adversely to these dyes, Dr. Ogden recommends washing new clothes before wearing them for the first time.[164]

When laundering our precious clothing, another area of concern can be static electricity and its resultant static cling. "It is usually caused from drying or wearing synthetic materials that collect electrical charges. . . . Some clothes made of these materials

---

[162] Lee, Michelle (2003) *Fashion Victim.* New York: Broadway Books, 240.

[163] Schwartz, Sara, "8 Underwear Mistakes That Are Bad For Your Health," Huffington Post. https://www.huffingtonpost.com/entry/8-underwear-mistakes-that-are-bad-for-your-health_us_5602b6dbe4b00310edf95264

[164] Clayton, Jamie Dalessio, "5 Ways Clothing Can Make You Sick," Everyday Health. http://www.everydayhealth.com/pain-management-pictures/ways-clothing-can-make-you-sick.aspx#06

will also start to cling to your legs as you walk, especially on days were the humidity is low or the air is dry. The skin becomes positive (+) in charge and the polyester clothes gain a negative (–) charge, thus causing them to attract."[165]

Most of the time, there is no serious harm, only an uncomfortable "shock" sensation and the annoyance of clothing sticking together. "However, the effects can be more serious under certain conditions. For instance, the shock can sometimes be sudden or painful enough to cause a physical reaction. This can cause problems like losing one's balance or spilling hot coffee on skin. In rare cases, this can affect cardiac pacemakers."[166]

In addition, the toxic chemicals used to alleviate the static are a great concern for many. "One common method to reduce or eliminate static cling on clothes is to use fabric softener in the washer, use dryer sheets in the clothes dryer or to use an anti-static spray on the clothes. Unfortunately, these are chemical solutions that may harm the environment and cause allergic reaction in some people."[167]

"According to the health and wellness website Sixwise.com, some of the most harmful ingredients in dryer sheets and liquid fabric softener alike include benzyl acetate (linked to pancreatic cancer), benzyl alcohol (an upper respiratory tract irritant), ethanol

---

[165] Kurtis, Ron, "Controlling Static Cling," School for Champions. http://www.school-for-champions.com/science/static_cling.htm#.Wfen4IgpBPY

[166] Martin, Chris, "Not Just a Tiny Shock: The Dangers of Static Electricity," Ultimate Mats Blog. http://blog.ultimatemats.com/2014/not-just-a-tiny-shock-the-dangers-of-static-electricity/

[167] Kurtis, Ron, "Controlling Static Cling," School for Champions. http://www.school-for-champions.com/science/static_cling.htm#.Wfen4IgpBPY

(linked to central nervous system disorders), limonene (a known carcinogen) and chloroform (a neurotoxin and carcinogen), among others.

"Since fabric softeners are designed to stay in your clothes for extended periods of time, such chemicals can seep out gradually and be inhaled or absorbed directly through the skin. Liquid fabric softeners are slightly preferable to dryer sheets, as the chemicals in dryer sheets get released into the air when they are heated up in the dryer and can pose a respiratory health risk to those both inside and outside the home."[168]

According to Dr. Michelle Schoffro Cook, author of *The Brain Wash*, there are several chemicals found in dryer sheets which have harmful effects on the central nervous system.[169]

Mike Adams, editor of *Natural News*, shares his concerns regarding the toxic effects of the perfumes found in dryer sheets. "When people use dryer sheets, they are coating their clothes with a thin film of artificial chemical perfumes. Just like other perfumes, a person's sensitivity to these perfumes decreases over time to the point where they don't even notice how potent these artificial fragrance chemicals are. None of this would be interesting if it weren't for the fact that these fragrance chemicals are extremely toxic. They are known carcinogens. They cause liver damage and cancer in mammals."[170]

---

[168] Scientific American, "'Greener' Laundry by the Load: Fabric Softener versus Dryer Sheets," Scientific American. https://www.scientificamerican.com/article/greener-laundry/

[169] Romero, Vanessa, "7 Toxic Reasons To Ditch Dryer Sheets," Healthy Living How To. https://healthylivinghowto.com/healthy-body-7-toxic-reasons-to-ditch-dryer-sheets/

[170] Ibid.

Donnica Moore, M.D. "also identifies dryer sheets as irritation culprits [for the vaginal area]. 'Many brands have a very high concentration of perfumes in them,' she states. . . . 'I recommend that women use hypoallergenic cleaning products as much as possible.'"[171] Raquel Dardik, M.D. concurs, recommending the milder the better.[172]

Non-toxic methods to reduce static cling include preventing dry skin with moisturizers, spraying the clothes with a light mist of water and running a metal clothes hanger over synthetic clothing before wearing.[173] Substituting ½ cup baking soda in the wash cycle instead of using fabric softener and ¼ cup vinegar in the rinse cycle instead of using dryer sheets may reduce static, as well.[174] (Be sure not to mix either with bleach, though, as resulting chemical reactions could cause noxious fumes.) Other options are to air dry synthetic clothing or only partially dry them in a dryer, thereby preventing or greatly reducing static electricity.[175] You can also try drying natural-fiber clothes separately from synthetic materials. The combination of

---

[171] Schwartz, Sara, "8 Underwear Mistakes That Are Bad For Your Health," Huffington Post. https://www.huffingtonpost.com/entry/8-underwear-mistakes-that-are-bad-for-your-health_us_5602b6dbe4b00310edf95264

[172] Ibid.

[173] Ibid.

[174] Zerbe, Leah, "5 Safe and Healthy Ways to Get Rid of Static Cling," Rodale Wellness. https://www.rodalewellness.com/living-well/get-rid-of-static-cling/slide/3

[175] Leverette, Mary Marlowe, "How to Get Rid of Static Cling From Clothes," The Spruce. https://www.thespruce.com/get-rid-of-static-cling-2146150

cotton and polyester is often the culprit behind static cling.[176] Some eco-minded individuals find felted dryer balls, made from felted wool, are their best solution to eliminating static, and therefore no longer need fabric softener or dryer sheets.[177]

When clothing is dry cleaned, chemicals are used as solvents to clean the clothing without water. "According to the Occidental College's Pollution Prevention Center, 85 percent of the more than 35,000 dry cleaners in the United States use perchloroethylene (or perc, for short) as a solvent in the dry cleaning process.

"Perc is a synthetic, volatile organic compound (VOC) that poses a health risk to humans and a threat to the environment. Minimal contact with perc can cause dizziness, headaches, drowsiness, nausea, and skin and respiratory irritation. Prolonged perc exposure has been linked to liver and kidney damage, and cancer. Perc has been identified as a "probable" human carcinogen by California's Proposition 65.

"Perc can enter the body through drinking water contamination, dermal exposure, or most frequently, inhalation. This is not only a health hazard and environmental justice issue for workers in the dry cleaning business, but for consumers who bring home clothes laden with perc. The U.S. Environmental Protection Agency (EPA) has found that clothes dry cleaned with perc can elevate levels of the toxin throughout a home and especially in the

---

[176] Scientific American, "'Greener' Laundry by the Load: Fabric Softener versus Dryer Sheets," Scientific American.
https://www.scientificamerican.com/article/greener-laundry/
[177] Romero, Vanessa, "7 Toxic Reasons To Ditch Dryer Sheets," Healthy Living How To.
https://healthylivinghowto.com/healthy-body-7-toxic-reasons-to-ditch-dryer-sheets/

The Healthy Clothes Closet

room where the garments are stored. Nursing mothers exposed to perc may excrete it in their milk, placing their infants at risk."[178]

Many clothing items labeled "Dry Clean Only" can be safely hand washed, or machine washed in a delicate cycle in a mesh bag. Check carefully with a published guide for specific advice. If our clothing must be dry cleaned, an option may be a "green cleaner" who advertises that they use non-toxic chemicals. Some use pressurized liquid carbon dioxide in place of perc to clean the clothes.[179]

Whichever type of dry cleaner is used, it is best to air out garments in a well-ventilated room or covered, outdoor location prior to wearing.

Dressing ourselves and our families in clean, lovely clothing certainly gives us pleasure. May we seek the least toxic products for our budget and lifestyle, and implement the healthiest laundering routine for our personal and our family's needs.

"Who can understand [all her] errors? Cleanse me from secret faults."
Psalm 19:12, NKJV

---

[178] Green America, "Green Dry Cleaning," Green America. https://www.greenamerica.org/green-living/green-dry-cleaning
[179] Ibid.

CHAPTER TEN

Complexion, Cosmetics and Colors

The Tenth Commandment

"You shall not covet your neighbor's house; you shall not covet your neighbor's wife, nor his male servant, nor his female servant, nor his ox, nor his donkey, nor anything that is your neighbor's."
Exodus 20:17, NKJV

Principle

Do not covet others' complexions, colors or cosmetics which are not health-promoting for you.

Our great God, "Who alone is immortal and Who lives in unapproachable light" (1 Timothy 6:16, NIV), was seen in vision by the apostle John on His throne surrounded by a beautiful, colorful rainbow (Revelation 4:3). Our Creator loves lovely colors, and He has planted in our hearts the same appreciation and delight.

There are so many wonderful colors to choose for our clothing! Most of us have our favorites we like to wear. When considering our health, there are effects of color that once known can positively influence our choices.

"Research shows that colours can have a psychological effect," states Jules Standish, author of *How Not To Wear Black* and a style and colour consultant for women. "When we look at certain colours it triggers neurological responses in the brain, and causes the hypothalamus gland to release hormones. Looking at warm, bright colours, such as red or pink, releases dopamine — known as the "feel-good hormone" — which can improve our mood, heighten the attention span . . . Cool blues, on the other hand, have been linked to the release of oxytocin, making you feel calm."[180] She therefore recommends those experiencing stress to wear blue.

"Bright red also triggers the pituitary and adrenal glands, which can lead to increased metabolism and weight loss, so it's great for a dieter", Ms. Standish states. "Purple is a calming colour — its pacifying effect makes it one of the best shades to wear when feeling overwrought. Research has found that we associate yellow with joy, so wearing it can boost your mood."[181]

The uplifting, stimulating effect of warm colors such as yellow, orange, red and gold have been recommended for those experiencing depression.[182]

"Gray is a neutral color that doesn't have a particularly strong effect on mood, except subconsciously," says color consultant Mary Ellen Lapp, author of *The Color of Success*. She warns against gray's "suppressive" ability. "If you wear gray all the time, you may not be the happiest person after a while," she says.[183]

---

[180] Standish, Jules, "Colours To Boost Your Mood!," Daily Mail, UK. http://www.dailymail.co.uk/femail/article-2864623/Colours-boost-mood-Dont-scared-clash-scientists-brighter-clothes-make-happier.html

[181] Ibid.

[182] Get Self Help, "Colour for Health," Get Self Help, UK. https://www.getselfhelp.co.uk/colour.htm

[183] Bowers, Elizabeth Shimer, "What Your Clothing Color Choice Says About You," Everyday Health.

Many believe that while red stimulates the appetite, blue can suppress it. One author warns, "We still need to be careful because wearing blue clothes always leads in time to fatigue, constipation and sometimes indigestion."[184]

Another consideration in choosing which colors to wear is to "select clothes according to a color palette that complements our own natural skin tone and eye and hair color—because the right colors help us look healthier, more attractive, and younger."[185] There are many resources to guide in color selection according to complexion. *Color Me Beautiful* by Carole Jackson is the classic book many use; however, there are other authors and personal consultants who can help determine one's best color palette.

Remember too that "your diet, lifestyle and general health can all affect your coloring. Let's consider what you eat. Many women are keen to try new foods, diet regimes and supplements. Some dietary supplements, whether organic or artificial, and fanatical diets can build up harmful toxins in the body that can affect the color of the skin as well as your health."[186] This brings to mind a dear friend who, in the interest of health, drank so much fresh carrot juice that her skin turned a definite shade of orange.

"Your lifestyle can also create 'high' or 'low' color. If hyperactive with stress regularly pumping your heart into overdrive

---

https://www.everydayhealth.com/emotional-health-pictures/what-your-clothing-color-choice-says-about-you.aspx

[184] Stein, Michael, "Color Clothes They Wear and Their Influence," Michael Stein. http://michaelstein.typepad.com/michael_stein/2011/06/color-clothes-they-wear-and-their-influence.html

[185] Spillane, Mary and Christine Sherlock (1995). *Color Me Beautiful's Looking Your Best*. Lanham, MD: Madison Books, 10.

[186] Ibid, p. 30.

you can look flushed and falsely 'warm' in skin tone simply due to high blood pressure or a raised pulse rate. When you are calm and rested you might look very different, less pink, maybe more neutral in skin color. Likewise when tired or lackluster from a sedentary lifestyle with poor circulation you can appear paler in skin tone than you might be if fit and active.

"If you are unhealthy at present or using prescription medication you might notice a change not only in your skin texture — the amount of dryness or oil secretions — but also in skin color. Some prescriptions can make you look yellow or olive in tone when you are usually a natural beige or even pink."[187]

If you are experiencing short-term complexion changes from health challenges, "put less of an emphasis on analyzing the color of your skin tone and more on your overall key coloring characteristic as well as your eye color and hair. Otherwise wait until you are fighting fit again and have regained your normal coloring before color analyzing yourself."[188]

Not only do we look healthier when we wear colors that complement our coloring but we also can be healthier. If we wear colors that make us look pale or washed-out, we may feel we need to wear heavy make-up.[189] A considerable amount of make-up often means excess toxins on our skin which are absorbed, contributing to our toxic load.

According to Kim Erickson and Samuel Epstein, authors of the book *Drop Dead Gorgeous: Protecting Yourself from the Hidden Dangers of Cosmetics*, there are many ingredients in make-up that have been shown to cause cancer in animals. "Coal tar colours, phenylenediamine, benzene and even formaldehyde are some of the

---

[187] Ibid.

[188] Ibid, p. 31.

[189] Ibid, p. 22.

toxins commonly found in shampoos, skin creams and blushers, they say. Hormone-disrupting chemicals, which could lower immunity to disease and cause neurological and reproductive damage, may also lurk in everyday cosmetics."[190] The authors warn their readers that chemicals from cosmetics can get into their bloodstream. "Hair sprays, perfumes and powders are inhaled; lipstick is swallowed; eye make-up absorbed by sensitive mucous membranes and others taken in through the skin."[191]

Among the cosmetic chemicals considered to be toxins are the phthalates. "Phthalates are used to make products more pliable and are found in toys, food, and some cosmetic products, such as nail polish and soap," says Adam Friedman, MD, an assistant professor of dermatology at Montefiore-Albert Einstein College of Medicine in New York City. . . . One recent study published in *Environmental Health Perspectives* found that women with high levels of phthalates in their urine were at an elevated risk for diabetes," as well as hormonal disruption in their fetuses.[192]

Other reported toxins found in cosmetics are parabens. "'They are preservatives used as ingredients in many cosmetic products, including deodorant, shampoo, makeup, lotions, and oral care products,' says Glenn Kolansky, MD, a dermatologist in Red Bank, NJ. 'They protect against bacteria growth.' . . . But a recent study published in the *Journal of Applied Toxicology* revealed that the

---

[190] Utton, Tim, "Danger That Hides in Make-up," Daily Mail, UK. http://www.dailymail.co.uk/health/article-108549/Danger-hides-make-up.html

[191] Ibid.

[192] Bowers, Elizabeth Shimer, "Is Your Makeup Killing You?," Everyday Health. https://www.everydayhealth.com/womens-health/is-your-makeup-killing-you.aspx

protection parabens offer against bacteria may come with a price: an increased risk for breast cancer. Researchers found that 99 percent of the tissue samples collected from women with breast cancer contained at least one paraben, and 60 percent of the samples contained no fewer than five parabens. Researchers suspect that the estrogen-like effects of parabens in the body may be partially to blame for the health risks they cause."[193]

Talc, a hydrous magnesium silicate mineral,[194] is a common ingredient in face powders, eye shadow and blush. "Talc particles have been shown to cause tumors in the ovaries and lungs of cancer victims. In 1973 the FDA drafted a resolution that would limit the amount of asbestos-like fibers in cosmetic-grade talc. According to the Cancer Prevention Coalition, no ruling has been made."[195]

Teenage users of makeup can face the additional risk of makeup-induced acne lesions. "Since teens often use makeup more heavily than do adults, they have a greater chance of suffering from skin problems. In addition, the pressure of body image and social status from their peers will prompt them to cover any blemishes with even more makeup. In turn, this action will worsen the acne, creating a harmful cycle of skin damage that may take months or years to reverse."[196]

---

[193] Ibid.
[194] King, Hobart M., "Talc: The Softest Mineral," Geology. http://geology.com/minerals/talc.shtml
[195] Ballestero, Shelly, "Are Your Cosmetics Making You Sick?," CBN. http://www1.cbn.com/700club/are-your-cosmetics-making-you-sick
[196] Alvarez, Manny, "The Damaging Effects of Makeup on Teens," Fox News.

An additional concern for teenage makeup users is the practice of sharing makeup and applicators with their friends without the realization of the bacteria and viruses that may be shared, as well. "This practice can lead to eye infections, cold sores, common sicknesses, staph infections, and even herpes."[197]

Solutions to the risks of wearing makeup include maintaining a healthy skin care routine in the form of a healthy diet and careful skin hygiene to reduce or eliminate the need for makeup. Additional recommendations are to avoid sharing cosmetics and applicators, wash applicators and brushes regularly, dispose of expired products, and be a label reader and avoid cosmetics with potentially harmful ingredients. In addition, websites such as safecosmetics.org are helpful for finding products which are free of toxic ingredients.[198]

For those with acne, determining food allergies or sensitivities may be helpful. A comprehensive book on the subject is *Food Allergies Made Simple,* by Phylis Austin, Agatha Thrash, MD and Calvin Thrash, MD.

One woman told me that when she was a young woman she was taught by the older women in her church to use hydrotherapy, in the form of alternating hot and cold wet wash cloths on her face, to stimulate the circulation and help prevent the need for makeup.[199]

---

http://www.foxnews.com/health/2017/06/16/damaging-effects-makeup-on-teens.html

[197] Ibid.

[198] Adams, Rebecca, "Why Your Makeup Is More Harmful Than You Think," Huffington Post. https://www.huffingtonpost.com/2013/08/09/makeup-harmful_n_3733000.html

[199] Robinson, Elizabeth, Personal communication, 1994.

As light entering a glass prism disperses into a myriad of spectacular colors, may the light of the knowledge of using color for our benefit extend into striking shades for our healthy clothes closet.

> *"Whatever is good and perfect comes to us from God,*
> *the Creator of all light,*
> *and He shines forever without change or shadow."*
> *James 1:17, TLB*

Conclusion

We have been on an amazing journey together, learning ten principles for a healthy clothes closet. It may seem we have reached the end of the path, but for some women it is just the beginning. It will take time for some of us to fully transform our wardrobes into a collection of health-promoting garments. The reward will be well worth it, not only because of experiencing better health, but also from the joy of being a positive example of healthy dress for other women.

Let us always remember that "in all respects the dress should be healthful. 'Above all things,' God desires us to 'be in health' — health of body and of soul. And we are to be workers together with Him for the health of both soul and body. Both are promoted by healthful dress."[200]

My heartfelt prayer is that we each may experience the many blessings of healthful attire. Amen [so be it]!

> *"Therefore I love Your commandments more than gold,*
> *yes, than fine gold!"*
> Psalm 119:127, NKJV

---

[200] White, E. G. (1905). *The Ministry of Healing*. Mountain View, CA: Pacific Press Publishing Association, 288.

Bibliography

Adams, Rebecca, "Spanx and Other Shapewear Are Literally Squeezing Your Organs," Huffington Post. http://www.huffingtonpost.com/2014/01/20/spanx-shapewear_n_4616907.html

Adams, Rebecca, "Why Your Makeup Is More Harmful Than You Think," Huffington Post. https://www.huffingtonpost.com/2013/08/09/makeup-harmful_n_3733000.html

Adams, Rebecca, "Why Your Purse Is Giving You Back Pain," Huffington Post. https://www.huffingtonpost.com/2013/12/09/purse-back-pain_n_4397727.html

Allen, Jane E. "Wardrobe Woes: Hidden Health Hazards of Clothing," ABC News Medical Unit. http://abcnews.go.com/Health/wardrobe-woes-hidden-health-hazards-clothing/story?id=15761031

Alvarez, Manny, "The Damaging Effects of Makeup on Teens," Fox News. http://www.foxnews.com/health/2017/06/16/damaging-effects-makeup-on-teens.html

Amazing Facts, *Amazing Health Facts!* (2009). Roseville, CA: Amazing Facts, Inc., 25.

Artisan Optics, "The Health Benefits of Wearing Sunglasses," Artisan Optics. http://www.artisanoptics.com/artisan/blogs/jill_a__kronberg__od/e_993/The_Eyecare_Corner/2017/3/TheHealthBenefitso fWearingSunglasses.htm

Ballestero, Shelly, "Are Your Cosmetics Making You Sick?," CBN.
http://www1.cbn.com/700club/are-your-cosmetics-making-you-sick

Best Health Magazine, "How to Choose a Healthy Handbag," Reader's Digest Best Health.
http://www.besthealthmag.ca/best-looks/beauty/how-to-choose-a-healthy-handbag/

Birch, Jenna, "These Are the Risks of Breast Implants, According to a Surgeon," Health.
http://www.health.com/mind-body/breast-implants-cancer-other-risks

Body Ecology, "6 Fabrics You Should Avoid Wearing and Why," Body Ecology.
https://bodyecology.com/articles/top_6_fabrics_you_should_avoid_wearing.php

Borreli, Lizette, "'Heel No Pain,' Foot-Numbing Spray, Eliminates High Heel Aches," Medical Daily.
http://www.medicaldaily.com/heel-no-pain-foot-numbing-spray-eliminates-high-heel-aches-lidocaine-hci-deadens-foot-pain-3-hours

Bowers, Elizabeth Shimer, "Is Your Makeup Killing You?," Everyday Health.
https://www.everydayhealth.com/womens-health/is-your-makeup-killing-you.aspx

Bowers, Elizabeth Shimer, "7 Surprising Benefits of Silk," Everyday Health.
https://www.everydayhealth.com/skin-and-beauty-pictures/surprising-benefits-of-silk.aspx#02

Bowers, Elizabeth Shimer, "What Your Clothing Color Choice Says About You," Everyday Health.

https://www.everydayhealth.com/emotional-health-pictures/what-your-clothing-color-choice-says-about-you.aspx

Butler, Alia, "The Importance of Positive Attitude to Health," Livestrong.
https://www.livestrong.com/article/126155-importance-positive-attitude-health/

Cancer Research U.K., "How the Sun and UV Cause Cancer," Cancer Research U.K.
http://www.cancerresearchuk.org/about-cancer/causes-of-cancer/sun-uv-and-cancer/how-the-sun-and-uv-cause-cancer

Cappelloni, Lisa, "The Best Activities to Do During Menopause," Healthline.
https://www.healthline.com/health-slideshow/ten-best-menopause-activities#2

Clayton, Jaimie Dalessio, "5 Unhealthy Handbag Habits," Everyday Health.
https://www.everydayhealth.com/pain-management-pictures/unhealthy-handbag-habits.aspx#01

Clayton, Jamie Dalessio, "5 Ways Clothing Can Make You Sick," Everyday Health.
http://www.everydayhealth.com/pain-management-pictures/ways-clothing-can-make-you-sick.aspx#06

Denka, Mary Brace, Personal Communication, September 13, 2017.

Doheny, Kathleen, "More People—Even Kids—Need to Wear Sunglasses," WebMD.
https://www.webmd.com/eye-health/news/20120517/more-people-even-kids-need-to-wear-sunglasses

Durning, Marijke Vroomen and Erica Roth, "Understanding and Dealing with Hot Flashes," Healthline.

https://www.healthline.com/health/menopause/understanding-hot-flashes

Environmental Working Group, "The Trouble With Ingredients in Sunscreens," EWG. https://www.ewg.org/sunscreen/report/the-trouble-with-sunscreen-chemicals/#.WdV- CNEpBPY

Fehr, Melissa, "A Guide to Activewear Fabrics," Seamwork. https://www.seamwork.com/issues/2015/01/a-guide-to-activewear-fabrics

Fitzpatrick, Kelly, "14 Creepy Ways What You Wear Could Be Hurting Your Health," Greatist. http://greatist.com/health/14-health-risks-you-might-be-wearing

Foot, "Foot Facts," Foot. https://www.foot.com/foot-facts/

Gary, Denetra. Personal Communication, October 13, 2017.

Get Self Help, "Colour for Health," Get Self Help, U.K. https://www.getselfhelp.co.uk/colour.htm

Greco, Jeremiah, "Wool vs. Cotton: When and Where" Orvis News http://www.orvis.com/news/products-we-love/wool-vs-cotton-when-and-where/

Green America, "Green Dry Cleaning," Green America. https://www.greenamerica.org/green-living/green-dry-cleaning

Groulx, Julie, "What Restricts Your Lympahatic Circulation?" MammAlive, The Healthy Breast Program. http://mammalive.net/mind-body-practices/restricts-lymphatic-circulation/

Hargrave Eye Center, "Health Benefits of Sunglasses," SlideShare. https://www.slideshare.net/hargraveeyecenter/health-benefits-of-sunglasses

Kime, Zane R. (1980). *Sunlight Could Save Your Life.* Penryn, CA: World Health Publications, 21, 31, 46, 117.

King, Hobart M., "Talc: The Softest Mineral," Geology.
http://geology.com/minerals/talc.shtml

Kiyak, E.K., "A New Nonpharmacological Method in Fibromyalgia: The Use of Wool," Journal of Alternative Complementary Medicine, NCBI, NLM.
https://www.ncbi.nlm.nih.gov/pubmed/19388862

Kurtis, Ron, "Controlling Static Cling," School for Champions.
http://www.school-for-champions.com/science/static_cling.htm#.Wfen4IgpBPY

Laskowski, Edward, "Can wearing a girdle help tighten stomach muscles?" Mayo Clinic Healthy-Lifestyle.
http://www.mayoclinic.org/healthy-lifestyle/fitness/expert-answers/flat-stomach/faq-20058288

Lee, Michelle (2003) *Fashion Victim.* New York: Broadway Books, 216. [Originally published by E.G. White (August 1, 1868) "The Dress Reform," *The Health Reformer.*]

Lee, Michelle (2003) *Fashion Victim.* New York: Broadway Books, 220, 221, 225, 240.

Leverette, Mary Marlowe, "How to Get Rid of Static Cling From Clothes," The Spruce.
https://www.thespruce.com/get-rid-of-static-cling-2146150

Life-giving Linen, "Scientific Details of the Linen Frequency Study," Life-giving Linen.
http://www.lifegivinglinen.com/linen-study.html

Life-giving Linen, "Underwear Testimonials," Life-giving Linen.
http://www.lifegivinglinen.com/organic-linen-underwear.html

LinenMe, "Benefits of Wearing Linen Clothes in Summer," LinenMe
https://www.linenme.com/news/benefits-of-wearing-linen-clothes-in-summer/

Main, Emily, "Your Purse May Be Contaminated with Toxic Metal," Rodale Wellness. https://www.rodalewellness.com/health/lead-and-purses

Marieb, Elaine (2006) *Essentials of Human Anatomy & Physiology*, eighth edition. San Francisco, CA: Pearson Benjamin Cummings, 488, 490.

Martin, Chris, "Not Just a Tiny Shock: The Dangers of Static Electricity," Ultimate Mats Blog. http://blog.ultimatemats.com/2014/not-just-a-tiny-shock-the-dangers-of-static-electricity/

Medical Dictionary, "Homeostasis," The Free Dictionary. http://medical-dictionary.thefreedictionary.com/homeostasis

Melissa, "How Is Silk Made?," Today I Found Out. http://www.todayifoundout.com/index.php/2014/10/real-silk-made/

Mercola, Joseph, "Sun Can Actually Help Protect You Against Skin Cancer," Dr. Mercola's Health Articles. https://articles.mercola.com/sites/articles/archive/2011/06/16/sun-can-protect-you- against-skin-cancer.aspx

Mercola, Joseph, "Women Beware: Most Feminine Hygiene Products Contain Toxic Ingredients," Dr. Mercola. https://articles.mercola.com/sites/articles/archive/2013/05/22/feminine-hygiene-products.aspx

National Cancer Institute, "Menopausal Hormone Therapy and Cancer," NIH https://www.cancer.gov/about-cancer/causes-prevention/risk/hormones/mht-fact-sheet

Mitchell, Heidi, "Do You Need to Wash New Clothes Before Wearing Them?" The Wall Street Journal.

Nedley, Neil, (2001) *Depression: The Way Out.* Ardmore, OK: Nedley Publishing, 88.

Norton, Rosemary, "Properties of Linen," Linen 4 Life.

http://www.linen4life.net/properties--care.html

Organic Lifestyle, "Organic Cotton—Why Bother?," Organic Lifestyle.
 https://organiclifestyle.com/organic-cotton/organic-cotton-why-bother?currency_code=USD

Pelletier, T.C., "Lanolin and Sheep's Wool Allergies," Ask a Naturalist.
 http://askanaturalist.com/lanolin-and-sheep%E2%80%99s-wool-allergies/

Peterman, William, "The Advantages of Cotton Clothing," Livestrong.
 https://www.livestrong.com/article/59826-advantages-cotton-clothing/

Positive Med, "Ladies Only: 5 Reasons Not to Wear A Thong," Positive Med.
 http://positivemed.com/2016/12/25/not-wear-g-string/

Robinson, Elizabeth, Personal communication, 1994.

Romero, Vanessa, "7 Toxic Reasons To Ditch Dryer Sheets," Healthy Living How To.
 https://healthylivinghowto.com/healthy-body-7-toxic-reasons-to-ditch-dryer-sheets/

Rossi, William A., "Why Shoes Make 'Normal' Gait Impossible," Unshod.
 http://www.unshod.org/pfbc/pfrossi2.htm

Schwartz, Sara, "8 Underwear Mistakes That Are Bad For Your Health," Huffington Post.
 https://www.huffingtonpost.com/entry/8-underwear-mistakes-that-are-bad-for-your-health_us_5602b6dbe4b00310edf95264

Scientific American, "'Greener' Laundry by the Load: Fabric Softener versus Dryer Sheets," Scientific American.

https://www.scientificamerican.com/article/greener-laundry/

Serena, "Wool Allergies: Their Causes and Effects," Love Knitting. https://blog.loveknitting.com/wool-allergies/

Shaffer, Alyssa, "Is Your Purse Wrecking Your Back?," Prevention. https://www.prevention.com/health/health-concerns/bags-and-back-pain-could-your-purse-or-handbag-be-causing-pain

Sheehan, Jan, "10 Tips to Keep Your Feet Healthy," Everyday Health. https://www.everydayhealth.com/foot-health/tips-for-healthy-feet.aspx

Skin Cancer Foundation, "Clothing: Our First Line of Defense," Skin Cancer Foundation. http://www.skincancer.org/prevention/sun-protection/clothing/clothing-our-first-line-of-defense

Skin Cancer Foundation, "What Is Sun-Safe Clothing?," Skin Cancer Foundation. http://www.skincancer.org/prevention/sun-protection/clothing/protection

Skin Cancer Foundation, "What You Need to Know About Clothing," Skin Cancer Foundation. http://www.skincancer.org/prevention/sun-protection/clothing

Sleep N' Beauty, "The Real Benefits of Sleeping on Silk," Sleep N' Beauty. https://sleepnbeauty.com/blogs/news/13894827-the-real-benefits-of-sleeping-on-silk

Son, SungMIn and Hyolyun Noh, "Gait Changes Caused By the Habits and Methods of Carrying a Handbag," Journal of Physical Therapy Science, NCBI, NLM. https://www.ncbi.nlm.nih.gov/pmc/articles/PMC3820208/

Sorenson, Marc, "Sun Exposure and Vitamin D Reduce Cholesterol Levels," Sunlight Institute.
http://sunlightinstitute.org/sun-exposure-vitamin-d-cholesterol/

Spillane, Mary and Christine Sherlock (1995). *Color Me Beautiful's Looking Your Best*. Lanham, MD: Madison Books, 10, 30.

Standish, Jules, "Colours To Boost Your Mood!," Daily Mail, U.K.
http://www.dailymail.co.uk/femail/article-2864623/Colours-boost-mood-Dont-scared-clash-scientists-brighter-clothes-make-happier.html

Stein, Michael, "Color Clothes They Wear and Their Influence," Michael Stein.
http://michaelstein.typepad.com/michael_stein/2011/06/color-clothes-they-wear-and-their-influence.html

Sullivan, Dana, "How to Lighten a Heavy Purse," Real Simple.
https://www.realsimple.com/health/preventative-health/aches-pains/heavy-purse#declutter-you-purse-daily

Susman, Carol, "Prevent Infections with Cotton Undies," Chicago Tribune.
http://articles.chicagotribune.com/2006-12-27/features/0612270268_1_cotton-underwear-vaginal-undies

The Fabric of Our Lives, "The Benefits of Cotton," Cotton Inc.
https://thefabricofourlives.com/learn-about-cotton/the-benefits-of-cotton

The Soxperts, "Best Anti-fungal Socks," Socks Addict.
https://www.socksaddict.com/blog/best-anti-fungal-socks/

The Wool Company, "The Benefits of Wool," The Wool Company, England.
https://www.thewoolcompany.co.uk/benefits-of-wool.html

34 Menopause Symptoms, "How to Dress for Hot Flashes," 34 Menopause Symptoms.

https://www.34-menopause-symptoms.com/hot-flashes/articles/how-to-dress-for-hot-flashes.htm

Thrash, Agatha, "Clothing," Uchee Pines.
https://www.ucheepines.org/clothing/

Thrash, Agatha, "Dress for Our Day," Uchee Pines.
http://www.ucheepines.org/dress-for-our-day/

Thrash, Agatha, "Healthful Body Temperature," Uchee Pines.
http://www.ucheepines.org/healthful-body-temperature/

Thrash, Agatha, "Menopause Assistance," Uchee Pines.
https://www.ucheepines.org/menopause-assistance/

Thrash, Agatha, "My Experience with Dress Reform," Uchee Pines.
http://www.ucheepines.org/my-experience-with-dress-reform/

Thrash, Agatha. Personal communication, July, 1992.

Tierney, Emily and C. William Hanke, "The Eyelids: Highly Susceptible to Skin Cancer," Skin Cancer Foundation.
http://www.skincancer.org/prevention/sun-protection/for-your-eyes/the-eyelids-highly-susceptible-to-skin-cancer

Top 10 Home Remedies, "10 Foot Care Tips that You Must Follow," Top 10 Home Remedies.
http://www.top10homeremedies.com/news-facts/10-foot-care-tips-that-you-must-follow.html

Underground Health Reporter, "Fact or Myth: Are Clothes Made with Synthetic Fibers Toxic Clothing and Hazardous to Your Health?" Underground Health Reporter.
http://undergroundhealthreporter.com/toxic-clothing-synthetic-fibers-hazard-to-health/

UPF Clothing, "Sea and Sand Can Increase UV Radiation by 25%," UPF Clothing.
http://upfclothing.org/sea-sand-can-increase-uv-radiation-by-25/

USCF Medical Center, "Protective Clothing for Skin Cancer Protection," USCF https://www.ucsfhealth.org/education/protective_clothing_for_skin_cancer_prevention/

Utton, Tim, "Danger That Hides in Make-up," Daily Mail, UK. http://www.dailymail.co.uk/health/article-108549/Danger-hides-make-up.html

Wakhisi, Sylvia, "Why Tight Clothing Exposes You to a Serious Number of Health Risks," Evewoman. http://www.standardmedia.co.ke/evewoman/m/article/2000120472/why-tight-clothing-exposes-you-to-a-number-of-serious-health-risks

Webb, Irina, "A Quick Guide to Amazing Wool Health Benefits," I Read Labels For You. https://ireadlabelsforyou.com/amazing-wool-health-benefits/

WebMD, "Fungal Infections of the Skin," WebMD. https://www.webmd.com/skin-problems-and-treatments/guide/fungal-infections-skin#1

WebMD, "What Are Hot Flashes?," WebMD. https://www.webmd.com/menopause/guide/menopause-hot-flashes

Weil, Andrew, "How Dangerous is Hormone Replacement Therapy?," Dr. Weil https://www.drweil.com/health-wellness/health-centers/women/how-dangerous-is-hormone-replacement-therapy/

Weil, Andrew, "Menopause Symptoms and Treatments," Dr. Weil. https://www.drweil.com/health-wellness/health-centers/women/menopause-symptoms-and-treatments/

Weinert, Anthony, "'Heel No Pain' Lidocaine Sprain: Numbing Your Pain Doesn't Fix Your Pain," Dr. Anthony Weinert.

http://dranthonyweinert.com/heel-no-pain-lidocaine-sprain/

White, E. G. (1923). *Counsels on Health*. Mountain View, CA: Pacific Press Publishing Association, 599.

White, E. G. (1952). *My Life Today*. Washington, D.C.: Review and Herald Publishing Association, 145.

White, E. G. (1958). *Selected Messages Book 2*. Washington, D.C.: Review and Herald Publishing Association. 461, 470, 473.

White, E. G. (1952). *The Adventist Home*. Hagerstown, MD: Review and Herald Publishing Association, 25.

White, E. G. (1905). *The Ministry of Healing*. Mountain View, CA: Pacific Press Publishing Association, 127, 234, 288, 292, 293.

White, Ellen G., *The Review and Herald,* September 23, 1884 par. 5.

White, E. G. (1947). *The Story of Redemption*. Hagerstown, MD: Review and Herald Publishing Association, 46.

Woolmark, "Benefits of Wool," Woolmark.
https://www.woolmark.com/resources/benefits-of-wool/

Zerbe, Leah, "5 Safe and Healthy Ways to Get Rid of Static Cling," Rodale Wellness.
https://www.rodalewellness.com/living-well/get-rid-of-static-cling/slide/3

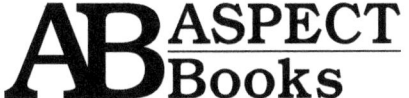

We invite you to view the complete
selection of titles we publish at:
www.ASPECTBooks.com

We encourage you to write us
with your thoughts about this,
or any other book we publish at:
info@ASPECTBooks.com

ASPECT Books' titles may be purchased in
bulk quantities for educational, fund-raising,
business, or promotional use.
bulksales@ASPECTBooks.com

Finally, if you are interested in seeing
your own book in print, please contact us at:
publishing@ASPECTBooks.com

We are happy to review your manuscript at no charge.

www.ingramcontent.com/pod-product-compliance
Lightning Source LLC
Chambersburg PA
CBHW051133160426
43195CB00014B/2451